Unrequited

ALSO BY LISA A. PHILLIPS

Public Radio: Behind the Voices

LISA A. PHILLIPS

Unrequited

WOMEN AND ROMANTIC OBSESSION

HARPER

An Imprint of HarperCollins*Publishers*

Portions of *Unrequited* were originally published in another form in the essay "I Couldn't Let Go of Him. Did It Make Me a Stalker?" in the *New York Times*.

HarperCollins books may be purchased for educational, business, or sales promotional use. For information, please e-mail the Special Markets Department at SPsales@harpercollins.com.

Poem on epigraph page reprinted from: "Dirge Without Music," *Collected Poems*, Edna St. Vincent Millay and Norma Millay Ellis (New York: HarperPerennial, 1981).

FIRST EDITION

Designed by Fritz Metsch

Library of Congress Cataloging-in-Publication Data has been applied for.

ISBN: 978-0-06-211401-3

15   16   17   18   19   OV/RRD   10   9   8   7   6   5   4   3   2   1

For Bill and Clara, who requite

I am not resigned to the shutting away
of loving hearts in the hard ground.

—EDNA ST. VINCENT MILLAY

Contents

Unrequited

Introduction:
The Unwanted Woman

ᴡ

I WOKE UP BEFORE DAWN. I WANTED TO
hold on to the blankness of sleep, but thoughts
of B. crept in too quickly. It had been a long
time since I'd been able to think of anything
else.

I'd imagined my future with B., and now
there was no future. Time moved forward
anyway, excruciatingly, every moment proof of
my abandonment. He wasn't with me, not this
minute, not the next. And he was supposed
to be. I knew he was supposed to be. He was
asleep in his own bed, a ten-minute walk away,
in his studio apartment on the ninth floor of
the Morrowfield, the tallest apartment building in Squirrel Hill, our Pittsburgh neighborhood. I couldn't reconcile the immensity of
what I was feeling with his faithfulness to his

girlfriend, a struggling actress who lived four hundred miles away, a woman he felt responsible for but didn't seem to truly want.

I hurried to the Morrowfield in the dim morning light. I stood in the lobby with its worn art deco tiling, slouching in front of the security door. I rummaged through my pockets, acting like a tenant who'd lost her key. Someone walked out and, asking no questions, held the door for me. It was easy to get this close.

I took the elevator to the ninth floor. I knocked softly on B.'s door. No answer. I kept knocking, letting the raps get a little harder, a little louder. The man in the next apartment opened his door. "Just checking to make sure it's not for me," he said.

"Did I wake you?"

"Nope. I get up early. Sounds like you're trying to get him to do the same." I nodded. "Well, good luck. Seems like a sound sleeper."

The man assumed I had every right to be there. I clung to that notion, his trust that I was just some tired student with bloodshot eyes waking up another for an early class.

I kept knocking. I counted, letting myself have five at a time until the total reached twenty, then thirty, then I lost count. I went out to the rooftop. It was November, two days before Thanksgiving, and gray. The wind whipped around me, and I thought back to that summer, of the warm nights B. and I had spent watching the sky, drinking bourbon and talking.

I went back and knocked again. I could do nothing else. Who would reject this kind of desire, desire that walks through security doors and knocks and knocks and knocks, refusing to go away? Isn't this what we all dream of, feelings so strong they allow us to flout the rules? This moment would be a story for later, when we told others how our romance started: "I couldn't get him off my mind, and one morning I just showed up at his apartment—"

B. opened the door a crack. He wielded a baseball bat in one hand and the phone in the other. "Phillips, get out of here," he said. "I'm going to call the cops."

I WAS IN love with an unavailable man, an old, sad story. When I first started to fall for him, months before, my feelings gave me pleasure and hope. I would wait for him, as lovers had waited for each other since the beginning of time. But as the months passed and he didn't come around, something inside me shifted. My unrequited love became obsessive. It changed me from a sane, conscientious college teacher and radio reporter into someone I barely knew—someone who couldn't realize that she was taking her yearning much, much too far.

How did this happen to me?

Years later, long after my obsession ended and I found someone else, married him, and became a mother, I promised myself that I would try to understand this bizarre transformation, which overtook me the year I turned thirty. I delved into the history and literature surrounding romantic obsession, courtship, and love, taking in everything from Renaissance medical treatises to contemporary advice books. I surveyed more than 260 women online about their experiences of loving someone who didn't love them back. Most revealing were the more than thirty in-depth interviews I did with women about their experiences of unrequited love. Their stories became the heartbeat of this book.

I also immersed myself in research in psychology and neuroscience, which confirmed what I observed all around me: It's common for women (and men) to be in unrequited love, and to have intense emotional and physiological reactions to it. They may obsess to the point of being able to think of little else. They may take the feelings out on themselves, acting in self-destructive ways. Or they may act out, emotionally and even physically, to hurt the person who's rejecting them.

Though unrequited love can get out of hand, it doesn't have to. I found in my interviews and in historical accounts of women's lives abundant evidence of the powerful *benefits* of unrequited love. It can move us in unexpected and important ways. And if we can gain enough distance from the pull of obsession to be able to understand it, unrequited love can be a highly meaningful state of mind, offering us insights into what we really want in life and love. Almost inevitably, it's *not* the person we've been fixated on.

WE LIVE IN an era of romantic practicality. The prevailing attitude toward the lovelorn, regurgitated again and again in formulaic advice books, is: If someone doesn't love you back, just move on. Yet research suggests that moving on isn't so easy. Unrequited love is a near-universal experience; in one survey, 93 percent of respondents had been rejected by someone they passionately loved. Both men and women experience unrequited love, and there is no clear evidence that one sex is more vulnerable to it than the other.

I decided to focus on women because society judges women in unrequited love more harshly. At the same time, it seems to understand them less. This tendency to dismiss the unwanted woman may come from the belief that women have more at stake in the mating game. They are the ones, with their time-bound reproductive systems, who are under more pressure to find a partner sooner, particularly these days. The median age of marriage is rising and marriage rates are falling; at last count, just 51 percent of adults eighteen and older are married. These demographic shifts have made finding a spouse in time to make a family together a competitive sport, with a thriving Dating Industrial Complex featuring speed-dating events and expensive personal relationship coaches. In this revved-up, commercialized, and markedly pragmatic mating arena, a woman preoccupied by impossible love is a pariah, indulging in a massive waste of time.

However, many women experience unrequited love when they're not in the dating market—they're already married, say, or have no intention of marrying or having children. Or they're too young or old to feel the pressures of the mating game. I believe there's another, more profound reason why we grapple uncomfortably with the idea of a woman who's consumed by unrequited love: There is something disturbing about the stubbornness of romantic obsession, about its unbridled conviction of rightness. The object of unrequited love doesn't choose to be loved. So unrequited love, even when endured in secret, without overt pursuit (the case with many of the women I talked to) is a form of rebellion—an uncontrollable (at least for a time) state of *I want* that persists no matter how the beloved feels and what common sense says. Unrequited love isn't sensible, obedient, or practical. It doesn't follow the rules.

We're far more comfortable, and, historically, more familiar with the idea of women as the *objects* of desire and pursuit. Self-help books advise women to yield to the fundamental male need to chase if they wish to find a committed mate. To win at love, women are supposed to make men feel as if *they're* in unrequited love, at least for a while.

This attitude targets more than just how women behave. We must not only refrain from pursuit, we must also tamp down what we feel. The typical prescription for getting over rejection and unrequited love is: Face the fact that he's "just not that into you" and forget about him ASAP. For today's woman, romantic obsession is dysfunctional and should be replaced by a relationship crafted by rational negotiation. Priscilla Chan may have moved three thousand miles to Palo Alto from Cambridge, Massachusetts, to be near billionaire Facebook founder Mark Zuckerberg, but not because she couldn't help herself. She made the journey only after carefully working out an agreement that every week he would spend "a minimum of a hundred minutes of alone time" with her and take her on a date. The arrangement apparently worked. After Chan graduated from medical school, the couple married.

The headline photos of Chan in her Claire Pettibone wedding dress contrast starkly with the dismissive stereotypes of women who get hung up on men who reject them. Unwanted women are tagged at best as pitiful neurotics whose lonely lives have become emblems of failure for their more disciplined and crafty sisters. At worst, unwanted women are freakish aberrations we're quick to call "bunny boilers," a term that alludes to Alex Forrest, the spurned woman in the 1987 film *Fatal Attraction* who leaves her ex-lover's family pet rabbit in a pot of boiling water; the expression has endured as slang for jealous exes and overzealous aspiring lovers. Alex—the "most hated woman in America," according to one tabloid cover—is one in a long line of sexy, relentless movie villainesses (*Possessed, Play Misty for Me, The Crush*) who tempt and then terrorize the men who spurned them. The media regularly feast on stories of real-life viragos: the astronaut Lisa Nowak; Betty Broderick, the divorcée who murdered her ex-husband and his new wife; and "Long Island Lolita" Amy Fisher, who at seventeen tried to kill her lover's wife.

The intrigue of these women seems to come from how extreme their behavior is. They allow us to indulge in illicit fantasy—for men, of untamed female desire, and for women, of unstoppable female revenge. Quite often they also make us laugh, becoming fodder for late-night talk-show jokes and snarky tabloid headlines. Female stalker films are often produced with an unmistakable camp aesthetic. When Beyoncé's Sharon tells Lisa, Ali Larter's stalker character in *Obsessed,* "I'm gonna wipe the floor with your skinny ass," it's hard not to laugh. But these cartoonish stereotypes give us little understanding of the painful experiences of women caught in the grip of unreciprocated love—and its impact on their targets.

Compare these stock impressions to cultural representations of men who yearn for a remote other. We know them historically as inspired and noble figures: the knight with elaborately romantic courtship rituals, the troubadour who sings of love and longing, the explorer who sets off into the wilds of Africa with his beloved's photograph wrapped in oilskin next to his heart. Great works of art have sprung from the heroic anguish of male longing: Dante's *La Vita Nuova*; Leoš Janáček's "Intimate Letters" string quartet; the many paintings and sketches Van Gogh made after Kee Vos, a cousin by marriage, rejected his affection. When men become aggressive and invasive in their pursuit of unrequited love, we don't mock them. We fear them, and we take action. In 1989 a wave of stalking murders of women in California—including the killing of television actress Rebecca Schaeffer by Robert John Bardo—shocked the nation and led to the passage of anti-stalking laws throughout the country.

Our understanding of when unrequited love is fuel for creativity, when it is romantically ardent, and when it turns creepy will always be clouded by some degree of subjectivity. Depending on the context, a love poem could be slipped innocuously under a beloved's front door or published in *The New Yorker* or become one more horror-show missive from an obsessed stalker. But when men are the pursuers, the line between romantic and threatening is more distinct. We don't question that men will want to initiate and pursue love interests, so we are more aware of the need for legal and social sanctions to keep these desires in check. This idea is rooted in what psychologists call the "chivalry norm": the notion that because men should be protecting women from harm, male aggression against women is a more serious transgression than female aggression against men.

Because women who yearn and chase are "out of their place," usurping a traditionally male prerogative, we're more confused about how to view women caught up in impossible desire and how to determine whether female pursuit has gone too far. We don't understand as much about the variety of ways women experience unrequited love and what light female obsession can shed on our understanding of relationships and gender. This book illuminates these issues. It explores the lesser-known, yet equally complex, cultural and historical representations of women in unrequited love. It addresses the psychology of why people become obsessed with an unwilling other. Throughout this exploration, I mine my own story and the stories of the many women I've interviewed— teenagers, college students, single women, wives, straight women, queer women, mothers, and grandmothers who, at some point, were too consumed by unrequited love to just "get over it." Some kept their feelings quiet, while some openly courted and pleaded. Some had a big crush that energized and inspired them. Others became deflated. Many toggled from euphoria to depression and back. Some became self-destructive, some invasive and aggressive. Most eventually came to understand themselves better. Several felt their obsession led them to make major changes in their lives.

What I've discovered through these stories is the importance of listening to unrequited love and seeking out its many possible meanings. I have come to believe that we must open ourselves to what unrequited love can teach us. What is our romantic obsession really about? What are we projecting onto those reluctant beloveds? What are we protesting? In other words, what is it that we're really yearning for?

THESE QUESTIONS TAKE on a different kind of urgency for women who end up behaving in ways they regret, like I did. Some of the women I interviewed became frightening and destructive. I don't intend to glorify unwanted pursuit or stalking, a crime that ruins lives. Inasmuch as I argue that unrequited love is potentially meaningful and life-changing, this book also delves into the ways romantic obsession can go badly astray, and how, and why.

The distinction between right and wrong in romantic pursuit can be particularly intricate for women. Women are far more likely to be the *victims* of stalking than the perpetrators. Anti-stalking initiatives are, like anti–domestic violence and anti–sexual assault programs, framed as protective of women, often with little or no mention of the possibility that men might be victims of these crimes. Even though more than one out of ten stalkers is female, we're reluctant to see women as aggressors who might pose a real threat.

Far more common are women who react forcefully to romantic rejection. Several studies of college students found that women are just as likely or more likely than men to resort to what professors William Cupach and Brian Spitzberg label "obsessive relational intrusion" (ORI)—ongoing, invasive, and unwanted relationship pursuit. ORI may fall short of the legal definitions of stalking, which generally entail a pattern of unwanted and threatening behavior that causes the target to fear for his or her safety. But ORI—what we might call "soft stalking"—still has a significant impact on its targets. These unsettling findings have remained largely under the radar. Society seems to be culturally blind to the reality of women's capacity for aggressive chasing, harassment, and stalking.

Research into male stalking victims shows that men who have been subject to relationship stalking by women don't believe they'll be taken seriously, and they're less likely to report incidents to the police. Men also face a "blame the victim" mentality. They're perceived as responsible for being stalked. Several men I interviewed said that when they talked about being the target of a woman's aggressive unwanted pursuit, friends criticized them for doing something to cause her behavior.

For years after I stopped pursuing B., I could not acknowledge that I'd gone too far. I blamed my behavior on him and his ambivalence. Even when I began to come to terms with my actions, my friends kept telling me, "Don't be so hard on yourself. He drove you crazy." But I'm certain that if I'd been a man, they would have had a far different reaction. They would have accused me of stalking—a word none of my confidantes used with me. We literally didn't have a language for what I'd done, just because I was a woman.

In the nearly twenty years since I pursued B., the idea that women stalk has become widely recognized—mainly in inconsequential ways. The voyeuristic opportunities of the digital age have turned "stalk" into everyday slang, its definition diminished in irony. "I'm so glad to run into you. I've been stalking you all day!" we might remark to a colleague, when all we mean is we've sent a couple of texts and an email. We can "stalk" online as much as we want, gazing undetected at photos and status updates. We can track someone's whereabouts on social media apps without taking a step. The term "stalking" has become a buzzword for the pursuit of a variety of female lusts. All-womenstalk.com is a cheery shopping and lifestyle site featuring articles such as "7 Tips on How to Accessorize Your Summer Dresses."

None of this constitutes real stalking. You can't be harassed without knowing it, so Facebook or Google stalking isn't really stalking at all—unless you're using these platforms to relentlessly message, bully, or threaten your target. Occasionally high-profile cases of true female stalking are received as novelty news, with plenty of victim blaming and sympathy for the aggressor. When Canadian actress Genevieve Sabourin was arrested for allegedly stalking Alec Baldwin, she asked as she was handcuffed, "Why am I being arrested?" The Huffington Post and other news sites were full of her defenders ("A female does not react in this way if there was no emotion, interaction or feelings. He's got $, she does not. . . . I feel sorry for this woman") and Baldwin critics ("That's what happens when you hit it a little too well"; "Alec is a sicko. Everyone knows it").

We need to reconsider our long-held assumption that when it comes to aggressive unwanted sexual pursuit, the victimized are always female and the victimizers are always male. Feminists and victims' rights groups have been trying since the 1970s to transform attitudes about sexual assault and stalking by educating college and high school students about sexual consent. In this book, I argue that we also need to remove what I call "the gender pass" for female aggressors: the mentality that, in short, lets them off the hook.

The very real potential peril of unrequited love does not have to undermine its power. Throughout this book, I defend the essence of unrequited love as a highly imaginative, life-altering experience that gives us insight about ourselves in a way that tamer emotions rarely do. The surge of feeling for an elusive beloved can be channeled in more productive directions. Pop superstar Lady Gaga once told *Rolling Stone* magazine that her yearning for a heavy-metal drummer who rejected her was key to her rise to success. Losing

him, she said, "made me into a fighter." Several of the women I interviewed testified that going through a romantic obsession brought
them to a place where they needed (and in retrospect felt destined)
to be—and wouldn't have arrived at any other way.

THIS BOOK UNCOVERS the many dimensions of women's experiences of romantic obsession. By offering an understanding of an
otherworldly and volatile state of being, I hope to ease the desperate bafflement felt by any woman who has ever been hopelessly obsessed. This book sheds light on the question: How could rejection
in love transform us so radically?

This is the book I wish *I* had when I was obsessed, the book that
would have helped me feel less alone. That said, this book presents
no easy answers to those of us who have been or are in unrequited
love—or are concerned about others lost in romantic obsession.
Rather, *Unrequited* explores the consequences and possible meanings of our feelings and actions. And it offers new possibilities for
our tortured hearts.

1

Do You Love Me?

THE ALLURE OF
UNSATISFIED DESIRE

❧

B. AND I MET DURING THE AUTUMN OF
my last year of graduate school, in a theater
seminar on tragedy. We were the students who
spoke the most in class. At times it seemed we
were talking mainly to each other, the rest of
the small class receding into the background.
I was attracted to him then, though he seemed
somehow remote.

At the end of the semester, he mentioned
he was dating another student, an actress in
the theater performance program. I didn't
know much about her except that she was a
Russian-born divorcée about to turn forty. B.
and I were twenty-nine. I also got involved

with someone else, a gifted short-story writer in his early forties. His career had started promisingly, with prizes and publications in well-regarded literary magazines. By the time we met, he was floundering. He juggled writing computer game scripts with short-term teaching gigs. He still hadn't sold the volume of stories he'd been working on since he was my age.

I looked past all that, and his two divorces, and fell hard for him. I had a weekend job as an announcer at the local public radio station, and he woke up early with me on Saturday mornings to keep me company at work. He teased me by calling me a "radio celebrity," even though all I did was push buttons and read a few minutes of news and weather every hour. Our relationship quickly grew serious, then unraveled just as fast. That summer, he went to New Hampshire for a month at an artists' colony and met someone else.

A few days after he broke up with me, I ran into B. I hadn't seen him much since we'd been in class together. We agreed to meet for a beer. He told me about the play he was writing, a one-woman one-act about Amelia Earhart. His girlfriend would perform it at a theater festival in the Berkshires. After the festival was over, he explained, they planned to part ways as friends. It was a fun relationship, but neither of them thought it should get serious. She wanted children and would soon be too old to have them. He wasn't ready. "I think I would like to have a wife, but I can't see it happening with her," he said. "I'm at least two years away from my Ph.D. I can't give her the stability she wants now."

I told him about my breakup. "At first it was so powerful to be so much younger," I said. "It seemed to redeem him, to bring him some sort of second chance at youth. But it wasn't real." I felt suddenly relieved not to have to play this role. I was glad to be spending time with someone my own age.

At the end of the evening, B. confessed that he'd had a crush on me when we were in seminar together. I walked out of the bar, the pain of my breakup no longer scalding. B. once wanted me from afar. His relationship was ending. Might he want me again? The idea thrilled me, and it was enough to lift me out of despair.

That moment, I realize now, was when I set into motion a chain of events that would lead to my obsession. I chose B. to love next, and I chose him specifically because he was not available. I was wounded, I told myself, and not at all ready to date again. The best remedy might be to spend time with a man who was not free to love me back.

I could have joined a bowling league instead, of course. But while bowling would be a mere distraction, B. gave me a sense of possibility that I badly craved. I would be good, I promised myself. I would not try to take him away from his girlfriend. Their relationship would move to its conclusion in its own time. I would have a chance to recover from my breakup. Meanwhile, B. and I would get to know each other.

For the rest of that summer, I got what I wanted. We took walks through Schenley Park, went to movies, and nursed milkshakes in the air-conditioned refuge of the Eat'n Park on Murray Avenue. On the rooftop deck of the Morrowfield, he played Willie Nelson songs for me on his guitar, singing the lyrics with a twang from his native Arkansas that was all but hidden when he spoke in class. He liked to call me by my last name. "Phillips," he'd bark playfully when I picked up the phone. I imagined he did so to emphasize the discipline of our situation. It seemed clear we wanted each other but refrained from doing anything because he was involved. We had, to quote the Louis Armstrong song, "a fine romance, with no kisses." I decided that was the best way to fall in love. In my past relationships, things had always moved too fast, too much intimacy before any real trust could develop.

THIS PARADOXICAL DESIRE—TO want someone you can't have—
isn't as strange as it may seem. Countless novels ride on the ideal of
the love that cannot be. It's a plotline that can stretch as taut as gut
strings on a violin. Whether it's played sweetly, sadly, or dissonantly,
we love to listen. Consider Edith Wharton's never-consummated
couples: Newland Archer and Countess Olenska in *The Age of Innocence,* Lily and Lawrence in *The House of Mirth.* There is always a
reason why one side of the couple can't return the love of the other.
Countess Olenska's failed marriage makes her damaged goods in
the eyes of New York high society, and Newland can't bring himself
to leave the far less enticing woman he is engaged to. Lily, with
her fragile orphan's status in New York City's elite, resists consid-
ering her friend Lawrence, who isn't wealthy, as husband material,
though they are clearly meant for each other. We rank these stories
among our greatest romances—yet beyond sporadic dramatic confessions, mutual love never fully develops in either tale.

When unrequited love does morph into reciprocated love, the
story usually has to end. Jane Austen's single female heroines spend
chapter after chapter weathering uncertainty and obstacles as
they figure out whom to love, and who loves them, until the plot
concludes with a round of marriage proposals, resolving all mystery. Nineteen thirties cinema capitalized on this theme in the
classics *Bringing Up Baby* and *Footlight Parade*, which end after
the heroine's unrequited love is requited at last. In our own time,
unsatisfied desire has propelled many hit television series to their
conclusion. In *Friends*, Rachel and Ross trade off hidden yearning for each other—and even parent a child together—before they
admit their mutual love in the last episode. *Gossip Girl's* entitled
Upper East Siders Blair and Chuck are obviously fated to be together, but during the show's five-year run, the two never pair up

for more than a few episodes at a time. The program was more enticing when they pined for each other, wrestled with jealousy, and flirted. They were two people who had everything except each other, until the show's last episode, when they hastily yet gladly married to avoid a criminal investigation.

Unrequited love is more romantic than mutual love and makes a far better story. Our earliest understanding of the idea of love emphasized the state of wanting, not mutuality or possession: In ancient Egypt, the hieroglyphic sign for love meant "a long desire." The state of not having, though on its surface an anathema in our rapacious consumer culture, is truly the essence of narrative. Whether the protagonist seeks treasure, a military victory, or a beloved, not having generates tension and suspense with the constant and pressing question: Will they get what they seek?

Once that question is answered, what happens next can't possibly hold the same drama. Passionate new love soon simmers down into the banality of a real relationship, with its petty arguments, trivial manipulations, and other small disappointments. In the concluding scene of *The Graduate*, the long quest to win Elaine by Dustin Hoffman's character, Benjamin Braddock, comes to a triumphant end as he wrests her away from her wedding to another man. The exuberant pair hops onto a city bus. They don't stay exuberant for long. Their smiles of victory fade to solemn, almost blank expressions. The newly freed lovers now must get to know each other not as glorious possibilities but as real people, about to experience the flawed and undoubtedly lesser reality of mutual love.

When I first fell for B., I was more than willing to wait for that flawed, lesser reality. I'd already had enough of it with my ex-boyfriend, who, once the early thrill of our romance faded, grew increasingly consumed by erratic work, disappointment over a broken book contract, and trading in his cantankerous BMW for a new Subaru, with monthly payments that would desiccate his already shaky budget. I wanted to relish my longing for B. It gave my life purpose. When I sat down to write, I wrote for him—to become the kind of person he would be proud to love. I read books and watched movies I imagined myself discussing with him (initially, I often did). I primped in hopes of seeing him. Just walking through the neighborhood turned into a sexually charged game of Where's Waldo? Is he there, in front of the Giant Eagle supermarket? Or huddled in a booth at the pizza shop? Or on campus, walking through the wrought-iron gates of the shadowy, cavernous ground floor of the Cathedral of Learning? I relished being in that story, that story of *not yet*. Whatever doubt or melancholy I went through in those early weeks was also sweet, my anthem sung in Lauryn Hill's throaty alto again and again on my stereo: *When it hurts so bad / Why's it feel so good?*

At times I thought B. understood completely what was happening, that we were creating this drama together. For my thirtieth birthday, he had given me the Milan Kundera novel *Slowness*, in which a character recounts the affair between Madame de T. and a young Chevalier in the eighteenth-century French classic *Point de Lendemain*. They spend an evening together, both knowing that the night will conclude with lovemaking. But Madame de T. persists in delaying the act. She makes small talk, she becomes angry. She walks with him through her courtyards and gardens, discussing her philosophy of love, sex, and fidelity. The conversation creates tension and suspense, all in the service of, as Kundera puts it, "protecting love" and turning desire into something memorable, a work of art.

THE IDEA THAT unrequited love can feel like an exalted state of being came to prominence in eleventh-century Arabia, in a blend of

Muslim and Platonic views about love and desire. Andalusian poet Ibn Hazm wrote admiringly of the lover's yearning to spiritually unite with the beloved, even as he cautioned against lustful physical consummation of the attraction. The lover, he believed, should be the slave of his beloved. He should address her as *sayyidi*—"my lord"—or *mawlaya,* "my master." The submissiveness bettered the lover, making him brave, strong, and generous. During the Crusades, these ideas spread to Europe, providing the foundation for what we now recognize as the courtly love ideal.

Like the spiritual longing Ibn Hazm described, courtly love entailed a strictly gendered division of responsibilities. Men loved. Women were loved. The vector of desire was supposed to go one way. Courtly love was never fully mutual and wasn't supposed to be consummated. In the troubadours' songs and poems and in medieval literature, the protagonist of the courtly love story had to either remain contented by the mere presence of his beloved, or suffer the misery of rejection.

Courtly love was *fin amour*—emotional, "fine" love—in contrast to marriage, which was not based on romantic feeling. Most unions were arranged before the intendeds reached puberty, and the purpose of marriage was to increase property holdings and sustain bloodlines. In courtly love, the besotted knight, who could not marry or own property in his prime soldiering years, politely yet fervently pursued his married lady beloved. He hoped for permission to kiss her hand or sit beside her for a few moments. The lady might express some degree of affection in return, or even allow him to see her naked body without touching it. Secret trysts did sometimes occur. But knights never expected to entrance a lady away from the bonds of marriage. Courtly love gave the knight a higher purpose in life.

For all its adulterous and subversive elements, courtly love served the needs of the court. The lady eventually had to spurn her knight's love, sending him, as historian Barbara Tuchman describes, into "moans of approaching death from unsatisfied desire." Then he would be off on his steed to perform heroic deeds of valor in her honor, seeking to regain her attention and advance his status in the court. The court benefited from a warrior who sublimated his desire into prowess on the battlefield, and the marriage of the lady and her lord remained intact, his bloodline secure.

But the idea that the unrequited lover had a mission that made his life more meaningful took hold in the medieval imagination. Unrequited love became the fashionable theme of the era, practically a cliché. From this cultural backdrop emerged literature's most renowned bard of unrequited love, the Italian poet Dante Alighieri. Dante first spotted Beatrice Portinari in 1274, at a flower festival in their hometown of Florence. They were still children; she was eight, and he was nine. But he knew he was fated to love her. As he recounted in his verse autobiography, *La Vita Nuova*, "Here is a God stronger than I, who shall come to rule over me." He pursued her in a wistful, boyish way, often going to places around Florence where he thought he might see her. When he was eighteen, she greeted him on the street, filling him with elation and providing the spark that night for the ultimate trippy unrequited love dream: A "lordly figure" held a naked Beatrice wrapped in a crimson cloth. He had a flaming object in his hand. "Behold your heart," he announced to Dante, then commanded Beatrice to eat it. Reluctantly, she did. The figure, weeping in grief, ascended with her to heaven. Dante woke up in anguish and began to write one of the many love sonnets he would compose in her honor.

Dante's unrequited love for Beatrice shaped his life's work. He was undaunted by the fact that they rarely saw each other, or that their parents had arranged for them to marry other people, or that she once got miffed at his lover's games (he pretended for a time to love another woman in order to screen his passion for Beatrice). The impossibility of their love stirred him rather than dissuaded him; he eventually decided he didn't want to try to see her, because he would just fall apart in her presence. He preferred instead to write "words of praise" about her. His passion endured after her tragically early death at twenty-four. In his masterpiece *The Divine Comedy*, Beatrice becomes an angelic Christlike martyr figure who guides him through heaven. His unrequited love wasn't really about a flesh-and-blood person. It was about devotion to an ideal, a way to glimpse the transcendent.

What Dante did with the idea of Beatrice underscores the fundamental narcissism of unrequited love. It is much more about the lover than it is about the beloved. It may feel submissive, but it is also egocentric—all about what extreme feeling for another can do to transform the *self*. As Dante writes in *La Vita Nuova*: "Thus pallid and void of all power, I come to behold you, thinking to be made whole."

Beatrice never made Dante whole by requiting his love. But his quest for wholeness through her gave him privilege—a subject to write about, a way to exalt himself through his feelings for a woman he barely knew. His desire was about asserting himself in the world through his fantasy love. As medieval studies scholar Howard Bloch put it, "The gaze is not upon the woman so much as on the reflection of the man in her eyes." What the beloved says or does to the lover becomes less important than what he can make out of the idea of her. In Dante's case, what he made out of Beatrice made his career and cemented his place in literary history.

Granted, the lady got a few benefits out of being adored. Scholars point out that in the glow of courtly love, women became more than a means to gain property and perpetuate a bloodline.

They could bask in the respect, compliments, close attention, and sensual pleasure of being adored. They had the right of refusal, something unimaginable in the marriage agreements their parents carefully negotiated. However, the object of affection in courtly love had no quest of her own. She did not have the privilege of asserting herself through unrequited passion. Being wanted is an inherently passive position. Her only privilege was the new view from her pedestal—but the surroundings hadn't changed. Medieval portrayals of women who *did* quest for impossible love make it clear that their infatuations were inappropriate, not enriching or heroic. In Malory's *Le Morte d'Arthur,* Sir Lancelot has no inclination to bask in the attentions of Elaine of Astolat. He chastises her for trying to make him feel "constrayned to love." Before she perishes of heartbreak, she arranges for her funeral barge to greet him at Camelot and prepares a letter explaining how she died. Her dramatic self-destruction is arguably a kind of masochistic self-exaltation—but a far cry (to put it lightly) from an ennobling quest or literary fame. The privilege of the unrequited lover was unlikely to extend to the medieval woman.

That's no shock, given the era. But as ideas of unrequited love and human equality evolved, this gender disparity has had considerable staying power. The nineteenth-century French writer Marie-Henri Beyle, known by the pen name Stendhal, took up the cause of unrequited love in postrevolutionary Europe. He was famous for being a serial unrequited lover, a man who, though he had a reputation as a plump womanizing dandy, glorified desire over consummation. His love affairs were rocky and transient; most were one-sided. He had a reputation for being sexually impotent, and the protagonists in his novels wrestled with timidity in romance. He never wed. In his autobiography, *The Life of Henry Brulard* (Henry Brulard was one of several pseudonyms he used), he took stock of all his loves and proclaimed that "my victories . . . did not bring me a pleasure even half as great as the deep sorrow caused me by my defeats." Unrequited love, for Stendhal, was a vital experience. He saw himself as picking up where courtly love left off. He may have begged his lovers to let him sit beside them, but he was just as enamored with the effects of *not* being with them; absence fueled his longing and imagination.

As he wrestled with his fiercest and longest passion, for Countess Mathilde Dembowski, he wrote *On Love*, the treatise that would ensure his place in history with its apt and poetic description of how passionate love affects the way the lover sees the beloved— and how the lover experiences the world. He called the process "crystallization":

> At the salt mines of Salzburg a branch stripped of its leaves by winter is thrown into the abandoned depths of the mine; taken out two or three months later it is covered with brilliant crystals; the smallest twigs, those no stouter than the leg of a sparrow, are arrayed with an infinity of sparkling, dazzling diamonds; it is impossible to recognize the original branch.
>
> I call crystallization the operation of the mind which, from everything which is presented to it, draws the conclusion that there are new perfections in the object of its love.

The image Stendhal offers here is both magical and organic. The process of crystallization comes from nature. But the result is that the ordinary becomes extraordinary, and only through the gaze of the lover. Crystallization is a state of mind. It shapes the way aspiring lovers see not only their beloved but also the world around them. Love is "a new goal, to which everything is referred and which changes the face of everything," Stendhal wrote.

"Everything is new, everything is alive, everything breathes the most passionate interest." Love, he believed, allows you to connect more deeply with *all* that is beautiful in the arts, nature, and human emotion.

Stendhal allowed that women could love deeply and unrequitedly. He professed to admire their hearts, and he advocated for their "moral liberty." Women, he believed, were particularly vulnerable to love; they had "too much grandeur of soul to love otherwise than with passion." In principle, it seemed, women could be the desirers as well as the desired, the crystallizers as well as the crystallized.

But with limits. Stendhal held that the experience of yearning was a far lesser one for women. "A woman at her embroidery—an insipid pastime that occupies only her hands—thinks of nothing but her lover; while he, galloping across the plains with his squadron, would be placed under arrest if he muffed a maneuver," he wrote. As Christina Nehring wittily points out in *A Vindication of Love: Reclaiming Romance for the Twenty-first Century*, Stendhal saw crystallization as "ultimately *creative* business for men, and *pathetic* business for women. The girl who 'crystallizes over her embroidery' is a target for pity. The man who crystallizes on the back of his arching horse is an object of admiration. The girl is a fool; the man a tragic hero."

Women, therefore, should keep their mouths shut about what they were feeling. *On Love* advised women to remain modest, withholding, and mysterious. These behaviors, Stendhal assured, would trigger the male imagination, and that was the important thing. Modesty was the "mother of love" and the source of what he perceived as a woman's ultimate power: to inspire a torrent of male feeling. A woman's yearning may be as strong as a man's, but

Stendhal did not believe she should reveal it to anyone other than her closest confidantes.

And so we see a frustratingly familiar caution take shape: Woman, hold back, no matter what the tumult is in your heart. It isn't your place to court and persuade. You may call for your rights—except in matters of romantic pursuit. The deliciousness of unsatisfied desire, at least for the stricken male, depends on your reticence. A woman openly taking on the quest to win her beloved's heart means such missions, and all they inspire, are no longer exclusively the right of men. The main mantra of *The Rules: Time-tested Secrets for Capturing the Heart of Mr. Right*, the 1995 book that spawned the self-help literature division of today's Dating Industrial Complex, is little more than an airbrushed, soulless descendent of Stendhal's promotion of female modesty. The book and its many spin-offs preach that a woman must never initiate a romance with a man; instead, she should cultivate an air of coy evasiveness to fire up his primitive need to pursue. We may sniff that *The Rules* is outdated and discredited (after her divorce, one of the authors sued her cosmetic dentist, blaming him for ruining her smile and hence her otherwise *Rules*-solid marriage; she has since remarried). But the main arguments, repackaged every few years through sequels and updates, have had remarkable staying power: Don't initiate phone calls, emails, dates, or sex, at least for the first several months. Don't agree to a Saturday-night date the first few times he asks you out—it makes you seem too available.

It still seems to hold true that many women buy into a clear double standard when it comes to finding love. One of the women I interviewed had spent her twenties and early thirties in steady, long-term relationships she described as egalitarian. Then she moved to a new city and, for the first time in her adult life, entered the dating scene. "It took me a while to get it," she said. "I wasn't supposed to be the one asking for a date or even choosing the restaurant. And that's how it works."

Though the unwanted woman can certainly playact this sort of passivity, the experience of romantic obsession is not fundamentally modest. It entails a near-perpetual state of self-absorption: *I want*, no matter what I actually do (or don't do) to get what I want. That selfishness is exactly what permits those torrents of feeling, the brilliance of perception Stendhal described. It makes possible the privilege of unrequited love: the assertion of the self through the idea of the beloved.

UNREQUITED LOVE SHOOK Diane's[○] world when she was a twenty-one-year-old art student and, as the Human League song goes, working as a waitress in a cocktail bar. At the time, she was entangled in an on-again, off-again relationship with Jeff, a possessive and moody bad boy. He angrily confronted any man he saw her talking to and hunted her down if she didn't come home when she said she would. She'd get frustrated and break up with him, only to return to him later because she couldn't shake the attraction. "He was a fiery guy, and I couldn't get away from the flame," she said.

Then she fell into a Stendhalian swoon over Roberto, a Mexican busboy. They had exchanged only a few words, most of them having to do with clearing tables. He had a regal bearing. His face, with its strong Indian cheekbones, looked noble yet sweet. He was reserved and industrious. She thought she caught him looking at her with interest.

---

* Many of the names in this book have been changed to protect the privacy of the people interviewed about their experiences of unrequited love. In certain cases, other identifying details have been altered.

On the basis of little more than that, she began to feel they were destined for a great romance. She had no interest then in marriage, but she daydreamed that she and Roberto might move in together one day and build what she vaguely envisioned as a "nice life." What they needed first, though, was a common language. Once she could communicate how perfect they would be together, she was certain, he would love her back.

Roberto, remote and exotic, had become Diane's beloved, glittering as brightly as a branch from Stendhal's salt mines. Suddenly, she saw the potential to renew her surroundings and her life. She covered her living room in 1920s wallpaper patterned with huge white magnolias. She planted zinnias in her yard. The dirt was hard, anemic, and full of nails, which she weeded out as she dug. She stuck the seeds in swirling rows of polka dots, like a painting. As the flowers pushed their way up through the dirt, she worked her way through a Spanish primer. Sometimes after work she'd get up the nerve to perch on a barstool, swig a shot of tequila, and practice her Spanish vocabulary on the bartender. She stayed away from Jeff. "I remember throwing the phone down the stairs and saying, 'Don't talk to me!'" she said. "Roberto gave me a place to put my affection that wasn't Jeff."

By the end of the summer, she had a scrappy patch of zinnias in her yard that thrilled her. And she had learned enough Spanish to ask Roberto out.

They went to an amusement park. They rode the Ferris wheel and ate corn dogs on a stick, flashing lights and garish colors all around them. With the conversation constrained by shyness and Diane's halting textbook Spanish, the evening was an exceptionally awkward version of the First Date. After wandering around for a while, they sat down on a bench, and Diane summoned up the nerve to do what she'd set out to do. She told Roberto she was crazy about him.

He explained to her carefully that his plan was to go back to Mexico, select a wife from his hometown, and bring her back to America. Under no condition would he ever have a relationship with a *Norteamericana*.

"You don't want to even try to get to know each other better?" she pressed.

He told her no, that wouldn't be fair. Their date was over. A few weeks later, Diane took another waitressing job. It was too painful to keep seeing him every day.

On its surface, Diane's story is about failure: her wasted time and energy on a fantasy that came to nothing. That summer she'd lived her life for a chimera, a man whose face told her stories she had few means of verifying. The only thing she was right about was that Roberto did turn out to be noble—too noble to start a relationship with her, a woman he could not have a future with. But consider what happened to Diane during her summer of unsatisfied desire. The crystallized Roberto became a repository of possibility, the gatekeeper to what Chekhov called a "new and glorious life." While this life didn't come to pass, something else did. Diane seized the privilege of unrequited love: to view the world and herself anew, and to assert herself through the idea of a distant love. She could see her rundown apartment and gritty yard as a canvas full of potential. She could learn a new language.

In the short term, she told me, her efforts were laughable. She was thrilled when the zinnias came up, but "they looked like crap." And her first real conversation in Spanish ended in heartbreak.

But in the long term, Diane's summer of unrequited love changed her in deeper ways. "It began my sense of the way that you plan for life. You do one thing now so that something else happens later. But you don't really know where it will take you." Her careful plans that summer did lead her in new directions. In her career as a professional artist and educator, she's made use of her Spanish in several photography projects she's done with Mexican families in the Yucatán. And though she went back to Jeff for a while, Roberto remained a symbolic antidote to the "irrational and powerful" attraction she felt for Jeff. Roberto "wasn't needy. He wasn't calling me, dogging me, distracting me from my schoolwork. He seemed self-contained, safe," she said. "I'm sure it was also safe that he had no interest in me whatsoever!" Eventually, she shook off her pull to Jeff enough to move to New York and leave him for good.

Certainly Diane exoticized Roberto. His remote otherness was fuel for her fantasies. The less she knew about him, the more she could imagine him into being—and reimagine herself. But doesn't the beginning of love often work this way—with a longing to get closer to someone we barely know, someone we see as full of mystery? Even when we know the person better, or when it's someone culturally more like ourselves, we have to endure plenty of unanswered questions: In love, what will he be like? What will *I* become? We use the unknown other to feed a dream of our own self. The beloved represents the blissfully perfect existence the aspiring lover wishes to have—what forensic psychologist J. Reid Meloy calls a "narcissistic linking fantasy," a common element in the passionate beginnings of love: "You feel like you've never felt this way before, that this is the most special relationship, that you share an idealized sense of a future together."

In the first swell of attraction, we are all unrequited lovers, uncertain whether our feelings will be returned. In this uncertainty, we give tremendous power to the beloved. Our feeling for him unifies our lives, defines us, infuses our view of the world. Our passion organizes our lives, thoughts, and actions. We're preoccupied with the question: Do you love me? The stakes in the answer are very high. Social psychologist Sharon Brehm calls passionate love a force that gives us the capacity to imagine a "future state of perfect happiness." When we dream of uniting with our beloved, we dream of an emotional utopia. We dream that love will complete us. In Plato's *Symposium,* one of our oldest written explorations of the nature of love, Aristophanes proposed that primeval man was once round, with four hands and four feet. But these early beings misbehaved, and Zeus punished them for their impudence by cutting them in two and sending the pieces off separately into the ether. Thus did life's quest become a reunion with the missing other half—a dream of oneness through love that emerges in some form across world cultures and religions. Unsatisfied desire allows us to imagine we have found the one who will make us whole, because we haven't yet tested the fit. The *not yet* relationship becomes strangely comfortable, at least compared to the risk of finding out your beloved's half-self won't conform to your own.

THERESA MET RUSSELL, another academic, when she was thirty-seven, on a Qantas flight out of Sydney. She was returning home to New York City after months of teaching overseas. She collapsed into her seat next to him. He had his head buried in a book. The flight was delayed. As the plane rolled from one position to another on the tarmac, seemingly aimlessly, he lifted his head and said in his broad Australian accent, "I think we're going to drive there."

That began an eight-hour nonstop conversation. They discussed their research and their jobs. Even though they were in different fields, they'd read many of the same thinkers. When they decided it was time to go to sleep, he offered her his shoulder to rest her head on. She was flattered but demurred. She was too excited to sleep. "I thought, 'I've waited my whole life to meet somebody I could have this kind of verbal connection with,'" she said.

He lived three hours away from her, which seemed to her a not insurmountable obstacle. They began an email correspondence. Their emails were long and detailed. They shared thoughts on books, movies, and what was going on in their lives. "It reminded me of the sorts of letters back when people wrote letters," she said. "It had a pen-pal quality with a romantic underlay."

At first she had no expectations. The emails, though enjoyable, were sporadic. She dated another man for a few months. That December, Russell wrote to tell her he would be coming to New York the following April to speak at a conference. "It would be great to see you again," he said. "Hopefully I'll look better. I'm sure I had drool all over my face on the plane."

The email triggered something in Theresa. "He wouldn't care how he looked if he weren't interested, I thought. And then it was like a cascade of feeling on my part. I got hooked into that zone of obsessing about him. He was the one I thought about every night."

The pace of the emails picked up. He sent her his photo and asked for hers. At times the emails were playful and fun. At times they were what Theresa described as "soul-baring." He wrote her long, heartfelt descriptions of his conflicted feelings about his mother, who was dying. Yet he made no plans to see Theresa before the conference, still a couple of months away. When she showed one of his emails to her roommate, she said disdainfully, "Look, he's not coming down to see you. He's just playing with you."

Theresa nodded, although her roommate's dismissiveness didn't seem quite fair. She had tried once to arrange a visit to see him, and it hadn't panned out. She hesitated to ask again, fearing she'd scare him away. Between the distance and the emails, she figured she would have time to let the relationship build. Their correspondence only seemed to get more personal; after his mother passed away, he sent Theresa the eulogy he delivered at the funeral.

The day of the conference finally arrived. She went to his talk,

dressed up and nervous. They had made plans to have dinner together. He casually suggested they pick up some takeout at Whole
Foods and eat it in Central Park instead of going to a restaurant. He
had a meeting at seven o'clock, he explained. This turn distressed
Theresa. After the months of waiting, he was barely giving her
enough time for a decent date, much less the long romantic evening she'd been hoping for. She tried not to let her feelings show.
They ate and talked. She asked him how he was feeling about his
mother's death. "It's complicated," he said evasively. They parted
ways before his meeting without making any plans for later that
night or the next day. She went home in tears.

An email from him arrived at ten. "I'm in bed with my novel,"
he wrote. He told her cordially that he had enjoyed seeing her.

Theresa was angry and confused. Who was this man who
wanted to relate to her only from afar, through his laptop screen?
In her reply, she confronted him: "Are you thinking about this as
something romantic or more of a friend?"

His answer: "Friend." He detailed the reasons why he liked her,
as if going through a list of criteria. She was beautiful. She was
smart. They were intellectually compatible. He'd had a nice time
with her that evening, but when she'd asked him about his mother,
he "just wanted to run."

Theresa puzzled over what had happened. So many signs of
promise were there. Others, oddly, weren't. She gave up on figuring Russell out—sexuality issues? Mother issues? The two inter-
twined? She would never know. She blamed herself for her own
bad judgment, for letting herself get so pulled in by an email exchange. She mentioned a divorcée she knew, a woman with few
romantic illusions and a surfeit of dating tips. "She always says,
don't sleep with a man for a few dates. Spend time getting to know
him, so you won't get hurt if it doesn't work out. That's what we

had. I never slept with him, but the effect was the same. I still got hurt."

Theresa had felt the verbal and written exchanges—all the sharing and confiding they'd done—constituted real intimacy, leading up to a deeper connection in person. Now she had to "change her definition of intimacy." For real intimacy to begin, she decided, a man had to do things for you. He had to deliver his *presence.* "Someone at my office told me, 'My rule is five emails, and that's it. If there's no date, it's over.'" Theresa was becoming everyone's poster child for the Single Girl Who Needed Guidance. She was pushing forty and still committing our era's worst sin: wasting time on yearning.

However much we might enjoy watching Chuck and Blair circle around each other on *Gossip Girl,* smoldering with sexual tension, in real life we contend with contradictory messages about unsatisfied desire. We live in a world with an unprecedented degree of disembodied romantic opportunity. Teens' first romantic relationships take place largely through texting, far more comfortable than the awkwardness of actually being together. Singles correspond online as a kind of relationship pretest to figure out if they want to invest the money, time, and emotional energy of getting together in person. The MTV series *Catfish* documents what happens when couples who have spent months or years smitten with each other online actually meet in person, with the slogan "Sometimes a little bit of fiction leads to a whole lot of reality." The program's hosts shake their heads as they read an email from Jesse, a young woman who wonders whether she should move to Alabama from her parents' home in Pennsylvania to be with a man she's corresponded with online for three years, even though so far he has avoided meeting or video chatting with her. "He just seems like the perfect guy for me," she gushes. Though some *Catfish* couples do find that their cyberspace love can thrive in the real world, Jesse does not, a fact foreshadowed by the many times the hosts harrumph, "There are so many red flags!"

There seems to be no real excuse for ignoring red flags, or skittishness, or getting lost in your imagination—or for accepting anything less than a partner whose needs neatly and scientifically conform to your own. The same online world that fosters obsessions with distant others also promotes a no-nonsense efficiency in matters of the heart. New romantic prospects can be tailored to our preferences, just like the boots we buy from Zappos, so we should get down to business and find what we want. Even the elusive idea of "chemistry" to describe that inexplicable sexual and emotional pull toward another has turned into a high-tech double entendre on Chemistry.com, an online dating site that uses a personality test (designed by biological anthropologist Helen Fisher) to connect people by personality type and neurochemical compatibility. So many options, and so much technology, should prevent a woman from getting hung up on anyone who is less than enthusiastic about a relationship.

Of course, it's much easier to point out the solution to the unwanted woman's problem than to ask what's so compelling about the *not yet* relationship. What Theresa told me was that the emails she received from Russell spurred her imagination, just as reading always had. "I lived in books when I was a kid," she said. "I have an excessive capacity to take fantasy over reality, to like the world of images and books and ideas more than the real world."

When we're caught up in unsatisfied desire, we can write the story of our love and, for a time, control it. This is fundamentally a creative act, often full of pleasure at first. We can be self-centered in a way that's impossible in mutual love. The situation is emotionally risky, because it's all about yearning to be together—yet being together means facing reality, which will probably fall short of the self-centered fantasy. But does that mean the fantasy has no meaning or purpose?

Longing may seem too complicated, too painful, too much of an anathema to accept in our instant-gratification, fix-it culture of Yahoo! answers and five-second movie downloads. Yet longing insists itself anyway. "Do you love me?" isn't the only question it asks.

"I AM ALWAYS in unrequited love," Katherine told me over her cell phone from her Massachusetts suburb. It was a weekend morning. Because she'd wanted to be out of earshot of her husband and two kids, she was in her car, parked in front of a café, drinking a cup of take-out coffee as it rained outside. The image brought to mind a clandestine meeting with a paramour. However, she was alone, and it was only her thoughts that were taboo.

Katherine, who is bisexual and in her late forties, is a well-respected educator. Her work and its impact on students, many of them from underprivileged backgrounds, truly matter to her; she is thorough and treats people with warmth and encouragement. She described to me highlights from the lineup of obsessive loves in her life: a boy who had a huge crush on her throughout high school and then backed away when she realized in her twenties that she'd finally fallen for him; the rakish coworker; the mother she came to know while their kids were in the same playgroup; the colleague she worked closely with. The unrequited loves start out as friendships and deepen quickly. "I love the process of getting to know another human being. You learn about their lives and have them learning about yours," she said. "It's a generative process. It teaches me things about my life. At that point, it's mutual. I connect with someone who wants to connect with me."

Inevitably, she begins to need more. She moves into a place, emotionally, where the people she's hooked on don't go. When she was in love with the mother, she wrote a note thanking her for her friendship. "I wasn't speaking sexually, but I made it clear the bond I felt was very strong," she remembered. "I think it threatened her. She didn't want to be that honest with me. And that was the moment when she began to pull back." Katherine calls that moment, which has happened with all her unrequited loves, The Withdrawal. The friendship doesn't end, but the air around it changes. The boundaries become clear and painful, thwarting the earlier exuberance. She tends to choose people who won't reciprocate.

She always tells her husband about her crushes, even though she knows it's difficult for him to hear. He doesn't try to stop her feelings or prevent her from being with the unrequited loves, though he may set limits—no nighttime phone calls, for example—if he feels her attention is drifting too often from the family. He makes sure to make friends with her beloveds. "If these people are not part of his life, they have to become a part," she said.

Her husband is a man Katherine has known for over twenty years. After nine years of somewhat rocky dating, interrupted by breakups and long separations, they married and had children. After all they've been through, she has faith that they will continue to love and support each other. "I have a sense of being loved for who I am in a way I've never felt with any of these other people," she said.

When I asked her why, with a husband she loves, she keeps opening herself up to these cycles of love and hurt and unsatisfied desire, she said it might be because of her father, whose love she never felt secure in.

There was another possible reason, a more existential one. "It's about the reality of our aloneness," she told me. "Ultimately, we all die alone. And at heart I'm a lonely person in the sense that even though I surround myself with lots of people and friends, I recognize that I'm alone, and that sense of isolation is hard for me." She spoke of the way her marriage—any relationship, for that matter—is like a Venn diagram of two overlapping circles. The marriage is the center. There are things she and her husband share and things they keep separate. "I get to keep intact who I am, and he gets to keep intact who he is, yet we connect, so it works," she said. "But there's a part of me that craves nothing but the unity, nothing but the whole. Nothing separate. Nothing off limits, nothing spoken but the truth."

Katherine's perpetual cycles of unrequited love seem an exercise in frustration. Her crushes never give her the experience of the unity she yearns for; they only bring her craving to the surface. As for many unrequited lovers, her fixation on her beloveds is about a need inside her—a need to stay in touch with the dream of perfect unity with another. When I told Katherine's story to a friend, she countered, "That's the kind of fantasy that my therapist would say was completely unrealistic and neurotic, and there's nothing good about it." This view is understandable and common. But it ignores the value of the emotional honesty of allowing yourself to feel love, even when it can't be returned. I admired Katherine for not pretending the pain of aloneness didn't exist—an angst most of us try to keep buried. Katherine wasn't shut down, huddled into her marriage as if it were the be-all and end-all of intimacy and addressed all of her emotional needs.

EVEN THOUGH STENDHAL didn't have women like Katherine in mind when he wrote *On Love* (he surely would have found her expressiveness immodest), his words allow us to distinguish what Katherine and other aspiring lovers do from the banal yet inevitable criticisms: How could she do that to her poor husband? Why would she put herself through all that? For Stendahl, the sweet spot of passionate love was in the quest. He had more faith in the vector of desire than in the consummation of it. When you walk up to the home of your beloved, he maintained, you don't really want the door to open. Face-to-face with your beloved, you might notice signs of your eventual defeat. You might say something stupid. Anything you do to try to let your beloved know how you feel takes you "away from the enchanted gardens of the imagination," he wrote.

I was a woman who walked up—or rather sneaked in—to the home of my beloved and knocked on the door until it opened. The enchanted gardens of the imagination weren't enough for me. I had to keep trying to turn my failure around, precisely because I perceived my position as the unwanted woman as failure. I didn't have to see it that way. I didn't have to give in to impatience. What Stendhal's words, and the stories of Diane, Theresa, and Katherine, suggest is that unsatisfied desire—those distracted, bittersweet days of seeing your beloved glitter with *not yet*—are worth something, even if they result in nothing. In the days of unsatisfied desire, we *did* feel more alive as we explored our new place for ourselves in the world through our desire for another. We planted zinnias, we opened up about our lives, and we daydreamed of an emotional utopia. We lived inside the suspense of "Do you love me?" and the myriad other questions that passion brings forth, questions about fear, aloneness, possibility, and what it means to be human.

The problems come only when we refuse to hear the answers.

2

Holding Out

FOLLOWING THE SCRIPT OF

UNREQUITED LOVE

❦

AT THE END OF THE SUMMER IN WHICH
I fell in love with B., he did not break up with
his girlfriend. After he came back from the debut of the Amelia Earhart play, he stopped by
my apartment to tell me. We sat at my kitchen
table, and I asked him if he still wanted to end
the relationship.

"Yes," he said. "But she didn't. We still
know where it's heading. We were not . . . We
were barely intimate."

"That's strange," I said. "The least you
could have done was fucked her."

"I didn't want to."

"I don't know what to do," I started to

chatter. "I know you haven't made any promises to me. But I—"
B. knelt in front of me with a resolved look in his eyes. I wanted to
turn my head away. I thought he was going to tell me he had to stop
seeing me.

He kissed me instead. We kissed for a long time, there in the
kitchen and then in my bedroom. I wanted to believe the kissing
was the end of the waiting. It felt like that at first, intense and sug-
gestive. We held each other tightly. I wanted to go further than
kissing, but he stopped me and left.

He came back a few days later for dinner. He was quiet, and
whatever conversation I could generate felt awkward. After we ate,
he told me he was tired and wanted to go home.

"What *are* we now?" I asked, though I hated to hear the words
come out of my mouth, petulant and demanding, so unlike the
easy fondness of before.

"I still have some thinking to do."

"Then why did you kiss me?"

"I thought it would help me decide."

"And me? Where does that leave me?"

"I can't tell you that." He headed for the door.

I grabbed his arm. He asked me to let him go. "You are a cold
man," I said, keeping my grip. I didn't understand how he could be
so distant.

"I am not a cold man," he said. I let go of him, and he left.

WHATEVER BENEFITS I had received from unrequited love lasted
only as long as my patience did. After B. kissed me, my patience
dissolved. The Kiss, after all, is what historian William J. Fielding called the "seal with which lovers plight their troth," an unmistakable turning point in the story of true love. For the unrequited
lover, The Kiss signals the triumph at the end of the long road of

forbearance, the moment when mutual love begins. Instead, the obstacles to my love became more and more significant, the situation more complex. If B. once intended for us to have a relationship, he had changed his mind, or his feelings for his girlfriend had become more binding than he'd imagined they could be.

What I hadn't thought of when I chose B., when I cast myself into this scenario of unsatisfied desire, was what would happen if I never got what I wanted. I was expecting the obstacles to be overcome, the suspense to be over, the story to conclude, the last episode of the television series to fade to black as my unrequited love downshifted to mutual adoration. It didn't matter if our love turned prosaic, as long as it was secure. I had yearned for him all summer. I needed resolution.

I didn't get it, but I didn't give up. There must be an explanation for how he was acting, I told myself. He must feel too guilty to leave his girlfriend for me. He'd told me all about his father, a wanderer and philanderer who died of a heart attack when B. was a senior in high school. It made sense that B. was terrified of walking in his father's footsteps. But I was sure that his relationship would end—he'd said, hadn't he, that it was bound to end? After he had some time to recover, we could be together at last.

My yearning in itself wasn't going to be enough. It had to be the means to an end. I would hold out, defeat the obstacles, somehow make this—us—happen. My determination felt renegade. In fact, the aspiring lover follows a distinct social script, as psychology researchers Roy F. Baumeister and Sara R. Wotman describe in *Breaking Hearts: The Two Sides of Unrequited Love.* They offer the real-life saga of Nicholas and Alexandra as a prototype for this script. When he was a teenager, Nicholas, a Russian prince and heir to the throne, fell in love with Alexandra, a German princess living in London. She spurned his advances for eight years and insisted she would never marry him. Finally, she sent a letter asking him not to contact her anymore. Instead of obeying, he traveled across Europe to convince her to change her mind. After two months of passionate courtship, she relented. The two became the czar and czarina of Russia, had five children, and shared a love so great that when they had to be apart, they wrote frequent love letters detailing their pain and longing. Their love lasted until they were executed at each other's side when the Russian Revolution brought down czarist rule.

Political upheaval aside, the outcome of the script is clear: If you persevere, you can win over your beloved.

Holding out for love can mean bold pursuit à la Nicholas. It can mean faithful waiting in the wings. It can mean carefully nudging a friendship toward romance. But the mythic script always ends the same way: Unrequited desire is a visionary force, driving both the hopeful lover and the beloved toward a relationship that is meant to be. The beloved's resistance, uncertainty, or obliviousness will one day yield. His marriage will dissolve, his girlfriend's appeal will fade. Unrequited love is love that is not *yet* returned. It is a caterpillar in a chrysalis, destined to transform into a butterfly and take flight.

As in the story of Nicholas and Alexandra, the classic version of the script features the male as the aspiring lover, the female as the beloved who comes around. The script has since become equal-opportunity, on heavy rotation in our collective psyche. At the end of the 1987 John Hughes film *Some Kind of Wonderful*, tomboy Watts hides her feelings for her best friend, Keith, as he pursues Amanda, one of the most popular girls in school. Once Keith and Amanda decide they're not right for each other, he finally notices that Watts is in love with him; he also realizes that she's the right girl for him. "Why didn't you tell me?" he presses her (in a line that alludes to Fred Astaire's famous unrequited love script-ender in *Easter Parade*: "Why didn't you tell me I was in love with you?" he queried his dancing partner, played by Judy Garland). "You never asked," Watts says. The couple kisses, and Keith gives her the diamond earrings he'd intended for Amanda. They walk down the street together, two working-class outcasts, obviously meant for each other all along.

When my daughter was seven, she and her friends favored the girl-power version of this theme in the video for pop star Taylor Swift's song "You Belong with Me." Still gorgeous behind comically huge black-framed glasses, Swift plays a geeked-out teen who has a crush on her next-door neighbor, a high school football player. They are close friends who exchange scrawled messages through their bedroom windows every night. But he's dating a bitchy cheerleader, also played by Swift, in vampire-dark hair and tight clothes that scream "fast girl." The geeky neighbor watches her beloved's rocky relationship from afar, knowing that he (as he confided in one of their messages) is "tired of the drama." She's too shy—and too virtuous—to overtly try to steal him away. But the song's chorus reveals her inner certainty and determination, cataloging all the reasons the cheerleader is wrong for him and all the reasons she is right: *I think I know where you belong / I think I know it's with me.*

The lyrics focus on her longing. Our heroine, like so many people consumed by a crush, never gets an answer to the question "Do you love me?" But the video my daughter and I watch on YouTube advances the story in keeping with the myth of perseverance. Geeky Swift appears at the prom, the glasses gone, her baggy T-shirts and jeans replaced with a virginal white gown, her beauty irresistible. Her neighbor pal promptly dumps the drama queen, who's dressed in a sleazy vixen-red dress. He gives the geek-turned-princess a deep kiss of approval. She was right. He *does* belong with her. Interestingly, Swift has since become one of pop culture's most derided unwanted women. She's been lampooned as predatory for turning her high-profile breakups into song material. At the 2013 Golden Globe Awards, comedians Tina Fey and Amy Poehler jokingly warned Swift to "stay away from Michael J. Fox's son," prompting Swift to parry back with the quote: "There's a special place in hell for women who don't help other women."

From Nicholas and Alexandra to the "You Belong with Me" video, we see the details of the unrequited lover's script emerge: The journey from unrequited love to real romance may be challenging, but with patience, hard work, or a combination of the two, you can overcome the obstacles and make it to your destination. You may struggle with doubt, but you should not give in to it. You have both your own happiness *and the happiness of your beloved* at stake. If Geeky Swift had abandoned hope and started dating a guy from the Math Club instead, she wouldn't have been able to attract her neighbor away from a girl who was clearly making him glum. Geeky Swift doesn't just win her man—she makes him happier than he realized he could be. And she overturns the faulty social order of high school, which dictates that the handsome jock will date the popular cheerleader, no matter what their true selves need. Geeky Swift's visionary unrequited love propels her to restore the jock to his true self, a guy who would have a much better time with a girl he can confide in and who shares his interests. The unrequited lover is the one who knows best, both for herself and for her unwitting beloved.

LIKE MANY WOMEN I interviewed, Janey, a twenty-one-year-old college student, is in unrequited love with a man who once loved her back. Their relationship ended not long after he moved to New York from Boston to go to law school. He confessed to her over Skype that he couldn't stop thinking about his own unrequited love, a high school girlfriend who dumped him suddenly and painfully and was now living in New York as well. "It's not fair to be with you and think about her," he told Janey. He also confessed that the comfort he felt with Janey wasn't really what he wanted, at least not at this point in his life. He was too young, he told her, to be experiencing such a smooth relationship. He felt like they had become a "calm, older couple."

Janey was waiting for him to come back. He wasn't far away anymore; she had transferred to a college in New York, a plan she hatched while they were together. She held on to the fact that, earlier in their relationship, they had been so in love that he spoke of marrying her. She told me she knew most people would say that staying attached to him wasn't "smart" or "good for her." She should shake him off and accept that their relationship wasn't meant to be. But these pragmatic options were simply not possible. Moving on felt like a lie. Their love, she insisted, was exceptional—a relationship in which they benefited from each other and loved each other unconditionally. "With him, I'm always learning, changing," she said. "We always have something to talk about. If we spent our lives together, I would never get tired of him." She told me that she couldn't help wanting to wait for him. "I've always been emotional and just care too much," she said. "I can't sit there and act like it's okay to not be in a relationship with someone I still love."

She hung on the words he'd chosen to explain why he was leaving her. "He's not saying he doesn't like me and doesn't want to be with me," she said. "That comforts me. He's just not looking for the thing we have at the moment. He wants something lively, passionate, reckless."

He also still wanted a lot of attention from her. He texted her often and saw her several times a week. They cuddled and sometimes spent the night together. "It felt like nothing had changed, except we weren't in a committed relationship," she said.

He was giving her plenty of reasons to hold out. He *was* still interested in her. He *did* want many of the things a committed relationship entails: closeness, constancy, physical intimacy. These signs sustained her, becoming the foreshadowing for the anticipated conclusion of her script: the restoration of their mutual committed relationship. Yet her daily reality was a kind of purgatory. However much Janey craved her ex's attention, the time they spent together stung. Right in front of her was a man she didn't truly have. Being with him as a friend painfully reminded her of how much she wanted him back. All the time she spent either with her ex or thinking about him kept her socially isolated and moody. Much of the time, she was miserable.

WHY DOES THE unrequited lover stay on script? Her perseverance often rests on whatever signs she can grab on to that the rejecter might change his mind. "The seeker has a confirmation bias, looking for positive signs and discounting the negative ones," Baumeister said. "If there's ambivalence, it's going to prolong the hope, because there are enough positives to seize on and overinterpret. The negatives you can brush aside." Janey's bond with her ex sporadically rewarded her desire for love, increasing his allure and spurring her to look for more. Behavioral psychologists call this "intermittent positive reinforcement." The impulse is similar to what prompts gamblers to keep placing bets, even when they're losing. All they can think is that the next time they put a token in the slot, they'll win, because sometimes they do. But in gambling and in love, this isn't a satisfying way to live.

What about her ex, with his mixed messages? There is no way for me to know what he really wants. Janey, like many of the women I interviewed, didn't want me to contact the object of her longing. He may not know himself what he's after. He may be too self-centered to realize how much the undefined nature of their relationship distressed Janey. He may be the kind of ambivalent guy others warn you to stay away from. Maybe he's a narcissist basking in her adoration, yet unable to get too attached. Whatever the case, the rejecter's advantage seems unjust. He is getting what *he* wants.

He may loom in our minds as a bad guy, even a sadistic tormentor. However, there's something else going on, something more basic than the endlessly intriguing but likely unanswerable question of what's wrong with the guy who doesn't want you back. Unlike the unrequited lover, a rejecter has no good script. He has an obligation to tell the unrequited lover that he doesn't feel the same way. Yet he knows that doing so will cause pain. The moral dictate to "tell the truth" dukes it out with another: "minimize harm." Either option leaves the rejecter open to criticism: How could he just break up with her when he used to talk about *marrying* her? How could he spend the night with her when he knows how much she loves him? No move he makes—except fully returning her love—will be right.

Pop culture sides overwhelmingly with unrequited lovers. It's their song that plays over and over on the radio, their plaintive expressions in close-up on the movie screen. A rejecter often doesn't know what to do or say. He may try to dodge the situation by avoiding the unrequited lover. Or he may go along passively with whatever the woman wants—putting off the moment when he'll have to say no, this isn't going to work.

There is much to dread about this inevitable moment of truth. For one, it hurts another human being. A rejecter may be asked to justify his feelings, while the real reasons would only compound the pain: You're so needy. You're unattractive to me. The sound of your laugh grates on my nerves. Your kiss made me squeamish. Often a beloved is at a loss to express precisely why he can't move forward beyond the simple, devastating truth: "I don't love you." A rejecter grapples with guilt and regret when he didn't intend any crime—he simply (just like the unrequited lover) *felt*. "They don't want to hurt someone or be the bad person, but they are thrust into a position where those are the main options," Baumeister explained. "It's like someone else is killing himself or herself and handing you the knife afterward and you have to take it."

And what a rejecter has felt—a lack of love—is precisely his crime. We're drawn to form close emotional bonds with one another. Attachment theory, first set forth by British psychiatrist John Bowlby in the early 1960s, maintains that human beings are social animals, born with a biological need to be attached to their caregivers. This need helps ensure survival. Babies who cry for their caregivers receive nourishment and other essential forms of attention: the cooing and talking that helps them develop language skills; the holding and sheltering that keeps them safe from predators. Research by psychologist Phillip Shaver shows parallels between attachment behavior in infancy and romantic behavior in adults: focused attention, holding, touching and other forms of affection, gazing into each other's eyes, and so forth. These parallels suggest that similar neural mechanisms are at work in both kinds of love.

In this light, someone who seeks love is naturally following the innately human quest for attachment. Someone who rejects love, Baumeister pointed out, is rejecting the opportunity to attach, turning his back on this most basic human desire to form relationships. The reason sometimes is that the rejecter is already attached to someone else. But often enough, the rejecter seems to prefer the unstable unknowns, the unpredictable state of being *unattached*. On a gut level, we can all understand this. Most of us reject arranged marriages, for example, as contrary to the natural impulses of humanity. We hold fast to the right to choose love. We don't want the choice to be made for us—and that's precisely what the unwanted woman does. She chooses the beloved, even if he's not interested or changes his mind. It's difficult to acknowledge the beloved's position as one he can't control, because he seems to have all the control. He is the one who shuns. If he refuses sex, his sin is even graver. Men are supposed to *always* want sex; as one male friend put it, "It's like when the apple falls into your lap. You're supposed to eat it." Of course, if he accepts sex despite his lack of interest in a relationship, he's toying with a vulnerable woman.

What complicates the situation even more is that we live in a historical moment with few reliable markers of relationship formation and commitment. We can insist, for instance, that Janey's ex is wrong for leading her on with all his attention—a romantic sin. You are not supposed to lead people on and then push them away. This unwritten rule consoles us. If your beloved is acting so sweet with you, he certainly doesn't intend to deny you the next steps: a date, a relationship, enduring love. Yet so often he will—it's a story I've heard again and again. We have a very hard time shaking off the sense that a certain kind of attention must lead to romance. We take an early expression of interest as an inviolable truth. Nothing our beloved says later, including "I don't love you," can have the same power.

Indignation about the person who leads a woman on is, to some extent, a vestige of earlier times, when mating rituals were more fixed. By the nineteenth century, arranged marriages in Western culture began to give way to the idea that marriage should be based on mutual love and free will, independent of parental supervision. But relationship building still relied on commonly understood signs of intent. Men sent flattering letters and sought private visits with women who caught their interest. Women responded by granting them time, offering encouraging words, and welcoming eye contact. Later in the process, kissing and heavy petting were seen as profound expressions of love and self-revelation, signaling a strong mutual expectation of marriage.

The rise of the dating culture in the twentieth century allowed for sexual intimacy that held no such assurances. Committed relationships evolved through dating, but they didn't have to. In postwar America, teenagers and young singles frequently "went steady," pledging loyalty and devoting all their attention to one person. Yet these "play-marriages," as cultural historian Beth L. Bailey calls them, were fickle. Breakups and new unions were so common that teenage girls at one Connecticut high school in the 1950s wore "obit bracelets," a chain of disks engraved with the initials of the boys they'd broken up with.

Yet steady dating still functioned in a set social order. It was the bottom of a hierarchy of types of commitment. Going steady might not pan out, but if you got "pinned" by a fraternity man, you had a higher-order promise in hand. Then came engagement and marriage. The protocol of what journalist and social historian Barbara Dafoe Whitehead calls the "national courtship system" was so widely accepted that the process of dating, falling in love, and finding a life partner in your twenties seemed natural and inevitable. As late as 1970, nearly 90 percent of women married by the age of twenty-nine.

Today, in the wake of the sexual revolution, the rise of birth control, and women's increasing economic independence, we are left with a mating system characterized by mind-boggling variety. There is still romantic dating and marriage, but more traditional relationships coexist with no-strings-attached sex, living together with no formal commitment, online dating services that provide an unprecedented wealth of new prospects, social media romances that boom and bust without the couple ever meeting in person. Whitehead points out that the new system is more inclusive and gives people more freedom of choice. Yet lost in the shuffle is "any coherent set of widely accepted practices or conventions" to that marriage or a committed relationship.

All these choices can have a paralyzing effect. A recent wave of studies on decision-making show that when we're confronted with too many varieties of jam or too many prospects in a speed-dating session, we become unrealistic, insecure, and less likely to make any choice at all.

In the current dating culture, the idea of "being led on" has become an anachronism. Where, exactly, could we expect to be led when there is no clear path to begin with? The liminal, neither-here-nor-there relationship is the perplexing default. We don't know if we're on a date or an outing, or how many dates mean we're now in a relationship, or whether sleeping with your best friend means you're "together" or merely "friends with benefits." We don't know whether we have grounds to be dissatisfied, because we have to consider what relationship expectations are acceptable. Are daily phone calls a right you can claim after you've slept together? Or only after you've agreed to be exclusive? Ambivalence thrives, with many relationships being neither *here*, firmly in the romantic, nor *there*, firmly not. This is particularly so for men, who can wait longer before they have to reckon with the question of whether they want to start families. The rejecter may not want you at all—or he may not want you back *as much* or *in the same way*.

I realize I'm asking for a lot here: an understanding of the position of the rejecter and his choices, which can, without question, be selfish, clumsy, and hurtful. My purpose isn't to let the rejecter off the hook. It's to show that the unwanted woman and her beloved are *both* self-absorbed, though we're more accustomed to using that label for the rejecter. They are living out two very different stories, with distinct sets of assumptions and expectations. The rejecter certainly should be aware of the potential impact of his erratic attention. But the hopeful lover should face the fact that the happy ending of the unrequited love script is *not* her rightful fate. In Janey's situation, the myth of her perseverance clashes with his illusion of endless possibility. She fixates on The One. Her ex-boyfriend, perhaps another kind of dreamer, believes The One is in the future somewhere or slipped by him in the past.

SONYA, A TWENTY-FIVE-YEAR-OLD design researcher, met Ryan through a mutual friend. The three met in Sonya's apartment before going out to dinner, and Ryan complimented her favorite chair. She was touched, because good design was important to her and it was rare for her friends to notice it. That summer, she and Ryan spent time getting to know each other, and she developed a "large burgeoning crush" on him. Then he disappeared. No one in Sonya's circle knew where he was. He didn't show up for his job. She was at a loss, at times disappointed not to see him, at times angry that he didn't tell her where he was.

Seven weeks later, he reappeared and told her what had happened: He had broken his neck in a bicycling crash. The injury, he added hauntingly, was to the same vertebrae Christopher Reeve broke when he was paralyzed in a horse-riding accident. Ryan had spent all those weeks recuperating in bed at his parents' house outside St. Louis. Knowing what he had been through erased Sonya's anger and amplified her feelings for him. "I felt like I wanted to take care of him," she said.

They went out a few times. They flirted. But he made no move to start a relationship. She began to believe he never would. At the end of the summer, a night out morphed into four straight days together. They holed up in her apartment, making out. "It was a whirlwind," she said. "Once it was moving forward, it was so fast that it was hard to believe it was actually happening. In four days I slept maybe ten hours. It seemed like we had this great connection."

Then he left and didn't call.

She waited. Waiting for the phone call (or the text, or the email) is a mortifying cliché of unrequited love. So many of us have been there. The whole situation feels like the worst injustice, worthy of R & B singer Macy Gray's helium-voiced protest: *We had such a good time / Hey! Why didn't you call me?* Even so, the unwanted woman can go a long way to rationalize the silence. There *must* be a reasonable explanation. He's lost his phone. He's busy. He needs space as he comes to terms with the momentousness of his feelings. Ryan, after all, had disappeared once before, and the cycling accident—which Sonya never could have suspected—justified his prior silence. Maybe there was something else that would explain what was happening.

Why didn't he call her? Silent avoidance might be a symptom of the rejecter's moral paralysis. There's another possibility: that he was in the process of deciding whether he wanted to move forward with a relationship. Sonya and Ryan were in a "reconnaissance dance"—the exploratory stage in the formation of a relationship. In this stage, potential couples or friends sample each other's company in an effort to decide whether they want to be together. The decision is based in part on an unstated cost-benefit calculation: what the relationship will give versus what it will take away. Sonya no longer needed to dance, so to speak. She knew she wanted to be with Ryan. She'd appraised him and determined that his insights, his intelligence, and his attractiveness would benefit her; they seemed worth the costs of holding out for him to respond in kind.

She also *bestowed* value on him. In loving him, she made him valuable beyond his objective appraised qualities. While appraisal asks, "What is the person worth to me?," bestowing value isn't evidence-based. It's more closely linked to the need for attachment, which isn't always rationally expressed. For most people, falling in love is something they can't control.

Chances are that Ryan and his ilk—The Ones Who Do Not Call—are having a very different experience of the reconnaissance dance. They are conducting a more detached cost-benefit analysis. And yet there's no good way for the rejecter to share this appraisal process with the prospective partner. It may be rude not to call after you've had an intimate four-day date—but what do you say when you *do* call? "Hello, thank you for necking with me for hours on end, I just wanted to let you know I'm still deciding how I feel about you and it isn't looking good"?

I had a disarmingly honest interview about the cost-benefit analysis with Lorne, a forty-seven-year-old entrepreneur living in a New York City suburb. In his twenties, he fell for a woman who confided that in girlhood she had been sexually abused by a relative. At first he was furious that anyone could have violated her in this way. He wanted to care for her and protect her. As he got to know her better, he realized that she wasn't the beautiful heroine he'd imagined. He saw her ongoing vulnerability and was frightened by what he perceived as her neediness. He told me he realized that he could not be her "knight in shining armor." The cost-benefit analysis he conducted no longer tipped in her favor.

He began to show up late for dates, or not at all, until she called him out on his rudeness and ended the relationship. Later, she tried frantically to get him back, distraught that a man she'd let herself trust had been so callous with her. He didn't relent. Her efforts confirmed for him that she was too much of a handful. He described his reaction as "she was nuts and I wasn't interested." Now he understands that he was too scared to be direct. He said that actually confessing how he really felt would have been "too emotional, too time-consuming," and he couldn't handle it.

Lorne's story is unsettling, not just because of how cowardly he was but also because there seems to be no way he could avoid being cowardly. The woman he was involved with deserved the love of a supportive man, but Lorne didn't have it in him to be that man. Faked love would not have done either of them any good. Being honest, the more ethical path, still would have caused her pain. And it's difficult to say which would be harder on her already deep psychological wounds: Lorne the irresponsible no-show, or Lorne the confessor, admitting his unwillingness to help carry her emotional baggage.

FIVE DAYS AFTER Sonya's long weekend with Ryan, he finally called. "I feel terrible," he said. "But this is over." The answer to "Why didn't you call me?" was belated but clear: He didn't want to continue what they'd started.

Sonya went through the rituals of getting over her disappointment. She immersed herself in chick flicks and tried to focus on starting her senior year. But she couldn't quite let go of all the significance she'd bestowed on Ryan. The day Sonya found out that a close high school friend had died after a long struggle with leukemia, she ran into Ryan. She embraced him. "I thought it was very significant that he was there," she said. "He'd shown up in that moment when I needed someone to be there." They met for dinner that evening. He made a confession quite similar to the one Janey's ex had made, admitting to his own preoccupation with The One Who Slipped Away: Just before his accident, he'd started to have strong feelings for a girl from his hometown. But after he was injured, she didn't call, and he hadn't heard from her since. He was getting over her, and that was why he couldn't have a relationship with Sonya.

For a while, she felt better. His rejection was no longer so mysterious. But their re-encounter launched another round of spending time together and flirting. They'd text each other often, competing in what she called contests of wit. She kept feeling that they were "building up to something," but that something never happened.

LAYING BARE THE dynamics of the interpersonal train wreck of unrequited love doesn't absolve anyone of responsibility. Ryan indulged his ambivalence in a way that seems unjust. We don't have to feel pity for the rejecter's moral quandary and difficulty in making decisions, particularly if he isn't treating us with dignity along the way. We just have to understand that the rejecter's challenges are significant and can cause confusion and pain for both sides of the unrequited love equation. The rejecter doesn't have to be a villain, or a broken soul who needs fixing, for the unwanted woman to face her real challenge: coping with the fact that she's not getting what she wants.

Yet the unwanted woman deserves some credit for her purposefulness. She is taking a stand amid—and against—the capriciousness of today's mating landscape. She is looking for a sense of power in a confusing situation. In the simplest terms, she has a clear goal, and she's doing what people working toward important goals do. They ponder and strategize. They face obstacles and try to remain patient. They take encouragement from signs of progress. They problem-solve. These qualities of perseverance are valued in most other areas of life. If we believe a goal is possible to achieve and we want it badly enough, we'll put in the effort over time to make it happen.

This dynamic helps explain the "motivational paradox" of unrequited love. Psychology researchers Arthur Aron and Elaine Aron developed the influential self-expansion model of love, which holds that being in an intimate relationship benefits us because it expands our resources, perspectives, and sense of effectiveness. We incorporate our partner's identity into our own and thus "expand" our selves. In unrequited love, we aren't getting those benefits, yet we persist in loving. "It's a paradox in that we're being motivated toward something that's not likely to be successful," Arthur Aron said. "You maintain a desire for something you don't expect to get. It's painful, and the more you try, the more painful it is."

What unrequited love *does* give us is a goal to pursue. The Arons found that the more unrequited lovers thought they had a chance of winning over their beloved, the more their love increased. And the more they valued the goal of having a relationship with the beloved, the more attached they felt. Both Janey and Sonya grappled with this potent calculus.

How is it possible to give value to a person who doesn't love you back? When I asked Sonya why her feelings had lasted, she said she couldn't quite shake her initial yearning to take care of Ryan, even after he rejected her. "There was a part of me that wanted to help him have better relationships," she said. "The caretaking impulse is a pretty big part of my life. I come from a family of social workers, and we have a long history of helping people. It was the way I was raised."

Behind Sonya's yearning, then, lay a larger reason. She needed to caretake. This need played out in her attachment to the idea of having a relationship with Ryan. Professors William Cupach and

Brian Spitzberg call this dynamic "goal linking." They describe the goal of having a relationship with the beloved (particularly when he does not want you back) a "lower-order goal," in itself not nearly as important as the higher-order goals it gets linked to, such as caretaking, happiness, easing loneliness, self-worth, the dream of a future with a loving partner. Lower-order goals can help us reach the higher goals, but the lower goals are supposed to be flexible and substitutable.

Goal linking psychologically binds the lower goal to the higher one. The beloved comes to represent something beyond himself and what's really happening. Sonya may have associated Ryan with her need for caretaking, but she couldn't take care of someone who didn't let her be close to him. The goal-linking theory helps explain why the script of unrequited love holds so much sway over the unwanted woman, even when it's getting her nowhere. Giving up on the beloved can feel like giving up on her most fundamental desires and dreams. It's the bestowal process on steroids. I remember all too well the way my world narrowed in the months I was obsessed with B. I saw in him my last chance for marriage and family. Looking back, I see how ridiculous it was to feel, at thirty, so dire about my future.

The concept of goal linking can help us see beyond that all-consuming matter of what the beloved is doing to us—how unfair, screwed up, and wrong his behavior is. "Rejection can be useful if a person can reflect on it," said Jacqueline Wright, an Atlanta-based Jungian analyst. "For example, what expectations did we have about the relationship? What unrealistic beliefs did we have about ourselves and the other person? This kind of reflection takes courage because of our tendency to take the easy way and blame a failure on the other person."

Even if we can't stop our longing, we can consider using the urge to persevere in another way: to better understand ourselves. What does the beloved *mean* to us? What ideas, needs, or dreams have we cast upon him? Then we might begin to understand what it is we're chasing.

MARIA GOT MARRIED in her early twenties to a man she never deeply loved. She explains it this way: She grew up in a traditional Catholic household. Her mother always told her to wait for a man to choose her. "Let them come to you," she used to say. When she was single, Maria spent her evenings hanging out in bars in the small New Jersey city where she worked. Around the time she turned twenty-three, she got tired of the scene. She decided it was time to get married and have children. One night she met Johnny. He spent the evening following her from one bar to the next. They started dating. He was good-looking, and he couldn't take his eyes off of her. He was also loud and boisterous. He smoked pot. He got around by hitchhiking. It was 1969, and plenty of young people were doing the same things. She shrugged off any doubts she may have had. Johnny had chosen her. She was ready to be chosen, and that was that.

She would spend most of their thirty-five years together trying to get him to, as she put it, "be good." She attended mass regularly and kept a strict workout schedule. She urged him to be more religious and take better care of himself. He shunned church, brought junk food into the house, and rarely exercised. He kept smoking pot. He got arrested for shoplifting. He was devoted to their son and loved his part-time work as a bus driver, even though it didn't bring in a lot of money. Maria's steady government job made her the family breadwinner. She was mad at him most of the time. Sex—which he seemed to want all the time—lost its appeal. She often endured it by fantasizing about other men.

When Maria was fifty-nine, Johnny died after a long bout with cancer. Several months after she was widowed, she struck up a conversation with Scott, a clerk she knew at a sporting-goods store she frequented. She found out that they went to the same church. "I thought, 'I could really get along with this guy,'" she said. "He seemed so nice, and I wouldn't have to worry about how to convince him to be different."

After a few more chats, she got up the nerve to ask Scott to go to Barnes & Noble with her. They browsed and talked. He told her that after he'd had a heart attack twelve years earlier, he'd changed his life completely. He stopped drinking and lost weight. He became so devout that he decided to be celibate until he found the right woman and married her. He'd been a bachelor all his life. All this made him thrillingly appropriate as a mate, though she worried that he might be holding out for a younger woman he could have children with. She was a decade older than he was. "The chances of me at this age finding somebody unmarried who is Catholic, interested in working out, and I'm attracted to him on top of it all? The chances of getting somebody better than that? Forget about it. I didn't think I would find anybody else who would be such a great match," she said.

For six months, they saw each other regularly. She usually initiated their outings. "I thought I had to be doubly aggressive because this guy was so passive and shy," she said. "I called him up. I thought, 'This is great.' It was a new experience for me to ask someone out. I was having the time of my life."

Their physical relationship was limited to hugs. She didn't want to have intercourse, but she wanted to be intimate with him. She mailed him a copy of a passage from one of her religious books about how it was morally wrong to have sex unless it was meant for procreation. It was her way of letting him know that she supported his decision to abstain, and that she planned to draw the line in the same place. He replied with a brief note: *Thanks for the material. I hope you find what you're looking for.* "In other words, a kiss-off," Maria said.

She couldn't accept it. She started to court him more ardently. "I thought, I never pursued a guy before in my life! And maybe that's why I never got the guy I wanted."

They continued to spend time together. She schemed about how she might make a pass at him. At home, she felt surrounded by memories of her late husband. It didn't feel right to be with another man in the same space where she'd lived for so long with her husband. Eventually, she got up the nerve to take Scott down to the basement, where the presence of her husband didn't loom as large. They fooled around. She felt aroused in a way she hadn't since the beginning of her marriage.

The next time they met, in the café section of a local supermarket, Scott was quiet and evasive. It was a warm fall afternoon, so she suggested they sit outside for a while before they parted ways. She went inside the store first to get some food and use the restroom. When she went out to the picnic table, he was gone. She looked for him all over the store. Feeling bereft, she drove over to his house. They had finally gotten close, she thought. She wanted to be with him even more, and he had abandoned her. She found him reading on his front porch. They took a walk and talked about their relationship. She asked him if they could see each other exclusively. He responded by telling her that he had promised himself he wouldn't do "wild things" anymore. He felt guilty about what had happened between them. She gradually realized he was letting her know that he didn't want to be intimate with her again.

She didn't contact him for four months. She cried so much she thought she was going crazy. "I thought, 'I have to see Scott, because I have a feeling that will make me feel better.'"

She started going back to the sporting-goods store. She went every Saturday afternoon for weeks. She lingered for hours to talk with him whenever he was in between customers. Every time she visited, she hoped he would ask her out, but he never did. One Saturday, she stopped by and found out from his coworker that he was going to be late that day. She did other errands. She kept checking back every hour or so to see if he had arrived. He never showed up. She was distraught about feeling so compulsive—and about the prospect that he might be avoiding her.

The following Sunday, she went to a later mass than usual. Scott was there. After she took communion, she walked up to him and shook his hand. She let herself look into his eyes for a few seconds, hoping for some sense of connection. His expression was blankly cordial. She went back to sit down next to her son. As the service ended, she tried to catch up with Scott, but he was out the door before she had a chance. She searched the parking lot for him and found his car. She saw him walking down the sloping lawn next to the church with a young woman in a miniskirt and heavy eyeliner. They were laughing together. The sight pained her. This was what he wanted, she thought—someone young enough to have children with. Then Scott caught sight of Maria. He turned around to walk in the opposite direction. She knew he didn't want anything more to do with her.

WHAT WAS MARIA chasing in this reticent bachelor? After spending so many years with a husband she was not compatible with, she wanted to be with someone who shared her values. She wanted a man she didn't feel she had to chastise all the time. These aims got linked in her mind to Scott. She couldn't imagine anyone else fitting the bill. And there was an even more important matter at stake. Her life had been marked irrevocably by the mandate that she wait for a man to "come to her" first. The man who did wasn't the right man for her. She had long berated herself for letting that happen.

In her widowhood, she had a chance to choose. Even though Scott broke her heart, the feeling of that momentary power remains indelible. "I'm glad I had the experience of being with the guy I was dreaming about," she said. "It wasn't right when I was married and having sex with my husband and really wanting to be in someone else's arms. This time I liked being in public with the guy I was fantasizing about. Choosing him was the best part."

It took her a long time to realize he wasn't choosing her in return. The pride of having spent time with a man she really wanted is mingled with the pain of facing his rejection. "I did everything I could, assuming he'd fall in love with me," she said. "I gave him too much. I didn't leave him any room."

Maria has come to understand that having choices in love doesn't mean she has to pursue them so single-mindedly. She also doesn't need to abandon the goal of real choice in relationships. She doesn't need to go back to feeling like the young woman she was forty years ago, ready to hand her destiny to the next man who chooses her.

3

Erotic Melancholy

LOVESICKNESS AS A LABEL OF SHAME

▾

NINETEENTH-CENTURY FRENCH PSYCHI-atrists called obsession *la manie du doute*—the doubting madness—because for the obsessed person, no reassurance is ever enough. What this felt like for me: The question "Do you love me?" went on repeat in my brain and became too loud for me to pay attention to much else.

I bought as many groceries as I could at the shop next door to the Morrowfield. I knew when B. was likely to be at the neighborhood café and peered at him through the windows, his head bent over a book, carrot juice and coffee at his elbow. I knew when and where his classes were. I cut a block over on my way to the bus, so I could walk the route he was likely to take. I kept my distance. I didn't want him to notice I was trailing him. Only sometimes did I let myself greet him face-to-face. It was natural enough for this to happen, as we lived in the same neighborhood and worked in the same building. I always hoped for news. Was he still with the actress? Did he still care about me? I didn't ask these questions, but they hung between us as we chatted politely. This stealthy tracking seemed the only thing I could do to feed the doubting madness. It kept possibility alive. If I hovered on the margins of his life often enough, one day he might return my gaze and announce that he was free to love me back.

This wasn't the way I was supposed to be spending my time. I had a one-year part-time teaching position, a job meant to allow me time to work on the novel I was writing. I wasn't able to concentrate enough to make progress on it, though. I was too obsessed.

Late one afternoon, I ran into B. I knew right away that something was different. He looked glad to see me, and it was easy for me to suggest that we have dinner together. Sitting across from me at the restaurant, he said he missed me. "I could just see this thing between you and me taking off," he said, angling his hand into the air like an airplane ascending.

My face flushed. My careful efforts were working, I thought. He told me that the only thing he needed to do was end his relationship properly, in person, when his girlfriend visited him the following weekend.

The weekend came and went. I waited until Monday evening to call him. She was still there. They had decided to stay together.

I fell into deep despair. I woke up each morning with a tremendous yearning I was certain I would not be able to endure. My days were shaped by my efforts to distract myself. I could not stay still. I swam lap after lap at the gym. I rode my bike for miles through the neighborhoods on the outskirts of Pittsburgh, sweating up the long, steep slopes of Bloomfield, Greenfield, Polish Hill. When it was too late to talk on the phone or exercise, I lay on the couch in my living room, too anxious for the small rituals of bedtime. It could take me an hour to bring myself to take off my shoes. I barely ate. I fell behind in my work, faking my way through classes I hadn't prepared to teach. Sets of student papers piled up on my desk. I could not quiet my extreme anxiety. I had been seeing a therapist, but she decided to leave her practice. I found another one, but the sessions with her didn't seem to help. And when she told me I was "going too far" in my efforts to win B., I canceled my next appointment and didn't go back to her.

I woke up one morning so overwhelmed by the prospect of facing another day that I checked myself in to the psychiatric ward at the University of Pittsburgh Medical Center. I didn't know what else to do.

You might say I was lovesick. The psychiatry resident didn't give me a specific diagnosis, though he told me in a matter-of-fact and not unkind way that I wasn't the first woman to check herself in over a guy she couldn't stop thinking about. He gave me a prescription for tranquilizers, which brought me stretches of relative calm. But the pills, which I allowed myself to take only occasionally, didn't cure me.

Lovesickness is a condition with a long and complex past. Since ancient times, we have seesawed between fearing lovesickness and being awed by it as an enchanted insanity, all the while dabbling with various cures. Today's scientific understanding of the brain chemistry of love and what happens when we lose it gives us more of a foundation than ever before to deem lovesickness a clinical condition, worthy of a place in the medical books and a pharmaceutically tailored cure. This sounds on its surface quite promising. I had, and still have, no objection to taking medication for relentless emotional pain. But as I delved into the colorful yet distressing backstory of lovesickness, I came to realize there were reasons to be wary of the disease model of romantic obsession. Historically, it has been used more as a means to control the unwanted woman than to help her. Lovesickness has been a label of shame, used not to heal but to put women in their place.

IN SECOND-CENTURY ROME, the famed physician Galen was summoned to the side of a woman described only as "Iustus's wife." We might speculate that Iustus was the one who demanded that she have medical attention, because she pointedly did not want to be cured. She was agitated and couldn't sleep, yes. But when the doctor arrived, she would not answer his questions and hid under the bedcovers. Galen came back to her home day after day, only to be dismissed by the maid, who told him that the mistress of the house did not wish to be disturbed. Finally, Galen managed to see her. Another visitor at her bedside happened to mention that he had just come from the theater, where he'd seen the dancer Plyades perform. Galen noticed a change in his patient's expression and complexion. He touched her wrist. Her pulse was irregular. Later, when he asked one of his associates to mention the names of other dancers while in the presence of Iustus's wife, her pulse didn't change. It wasn't until Galen was present for an announcement that Plyades would be performing that he caught disturbances in her pulse again.

Galen had his diagnosis: Iustus's wife was besotted with Plyades. It was the first documented instance of a woman being diagnosed with lovesickness. What this meant, under the Hippocratic system of the day, was that the passion Iustus's wife felt for the dancer had created an imbalance in the four essential humors, or fluids, of her body, causing her physical symptoms.

Iustus's wife may have been out of balance, a concept that foreshadows our contemporary understanding of the combination of hormones necessary for emotional regulation. More important, she was out of bounds. A wife's primary function in ancient Rome was to produce children, perpetuate her husband's bloodline, and make family alliances that would help him increase his holdings. The Roman man was defined through his property. The more land, livestock, money, and slaves he owned, the greater his status. The myth behind the founding of Rome, in fact, is a cautionary tale about the value of property over passion. In the story of Dido and Aeneas, Dido, a widowed African queen, falls in love with Aeneas, a Trojan hero who has accidentally landed on her shores in the wake of the fall of Troy. She becomes, as Virgil describes in *The Aeneid*, "wild with passion" and consumed by a "rage of desire." Aeneas loves her back—yet the gods swoop in to ruin the couple. His fate, they decree, is to create a new city in Italy. Dido pleads for him to stay with her, but he won't. She drags their bed and some of his belongings, including a sword she gave him, into a courtyard and sets them on fire. She climbs to the top of the pyre, falls on Aeneas's sword, and perishes as his ship sails away.

Dido's fate exemplifies the ancient Greek and Roman mistrust of passionate love as a "divine madness" sent from the gods, a threat to social order and progress. If Dido had succeeded in keeping Aeneas by her side, the myth suggests, then Rome, the world's first big city, would not exist. Her all-consuming passion was a threat to progress and greatness. In a similar fashion, the jittery longing that Iustus's wife felt for Plyades, who was likely a slave or a freedman, presented a threat to Iustus's hold on his property and the social order that protected it. An affair between his wife and the dancer would be adulterous, disreputable, and illegal. While the law didn't penalize men who cheated on their wives, wives who strayed lost half their dowry and were forbidden to ever marry their paramours. Under these conditions, the nameless wife's desire was an emotional rebellion against the rigid social order. She dreamed of a life in which she was more than property and a womb, a life in which she had erotic agency that reached across stringent class divides and defied the constraints of what was likely a less than satisfactory marriage. Galen's diagnosis took none of this into account. It reduced all her feeling, and its social context, into an illness to be cured.

Galen, who detailed the case in *On Prognosis*, his major work, did not describe how the lovesickness of Iustus's wife was resolved. At the time, the standard cure for lovesickness was "therapeutic intercourse," ideally after you'd married the love object. If marriage wasn't possible, available surrogates such as prostitutes, slaves, or widows might do—but these were options available only to men. Even the marriage cure probably panned out only in instances when a girl's lovesickness was over someone her father happened to find suitable husband material, an unlikely situation when girls were married off in their teens.

While the prevailing attitude toward female lovesickness reinforced women's constrained role in ancient Rome, male lovesickness was seen as a force that could successfully *transform* the social order. Galen's pulse test for diagnosing lovesickness was based on the approach used by the physician Erasistratus on Antiochus, the son of Seleucus, the king of Syria. Antiochus fell in love with his stepmother, Stratonice. His secret longing made him so miserable that he intended to starve himself to death. To figure out what ailed Antiochus, Erasistratus kept a close watch on how the prince reacted to the beauties of the court. When Stratonice entered the room, Erasistratus watched Antiochus turn pale, stammer, then flush red. The doctor felt Antiochus's heart and found it palpitating wildly. Antiochus's love, like the desire of Iustus's wife, was transgressive and seemingly impossible, as Stratonice belonged to his father, the king. Yet amazingly, once the physician told King Seleucus what was wrong with Antiochus, the king ended his marriage. He gave his wife to his son and made the couple the rulers of what was then known as Upper Asia. Antiochus was instantly cured.

The stories of Antiochus and of Iustus's wife are repeated in medical treatises and literature from ancient times through the Renaissance. Their contrasting fates—the prince who gets what he wants and the nameless wife who doesn't—underscore a double standard for male and female victims of lovesickness. Antiochus's lovesickness was righteous, the cure increasing his personal power and justifying the demise of his father's royal union. Iustus's wife gets nothing but a diagnosis, a label put on her insubordinate heart. For men, lovesickness had heroic and erotic power. For women, the disease emphasized their degradation.

These ancient meanings carried considerable weight as lovesickness became more entrenched as a disease category. In the early Middle Ages, Arabic physicians saw the main cause of lovesickness to be the buildup of *sperma*, a substance that, in the medical understanding of the day, both men's and women's bodies produced. The cure remained the same: intercourse, if possible, with the love object; if not, with a prostitute or a slave. This view spread to Europe via Constantine, a North African physician who translated Arabic medical handbooks into Latin. For a while, European physicians conveniently ignored the question of where women fit in to the disease model. Lovesickness became known as *amor hereos*, a term that translates as "heroic love" but has more to do with the social status of the lover than his courage. *Amor hereos* was a disease of entitlement, primarily affecting noblemen. The noblemen's symptoms—obsessive thinking, loss of appetite, heart palpitations, and the like—were not much different from those of the knights and troubadours whose obsession inspired them to feats of bravery, poetry, and song. The noblemen, though, lived lives of comfort and leisure and didn't have to sublimate their desires into making war or art.

By the thirteenth century, more women—also typically of the entitled classes—were seeking medical attention for the symptoms of lovesickness. Discussions of "erotic melancholy" and "uterine fury" began to show up in the medical literature. The increasing familiarity of female lovesickness in the late Middle Ages and Renaissance did not make it any more honorable for women. Uterine fury described a kind of bodily rage, a loss of control and decorum. It was a condition of shame and vulnerability, an indication that the sufferer needed marital connection.

In *A Treatise on Lovesickness*, published in 1623, physician Jacques Ferrand warned women that the excessive lust of lovesickness would leave them vulnerable to dishonor. He saw women as more susceptible to lovesickness than men, owing to the presence of female "spermatic vessels" (what we now call fallopian tubes) inside the main cavity of the body, too near the repositories of imagination and judgment; in men, these vessels were farther away and less likely to interfere with rationality. The ideal cure for women, as for men, was marriage and marital sex.

If marriage couldn't calm a woman's uterine fury, Ferrand believed, the prospect of being what we would now call "slut-shamed" might. He compared the lovesick woman's plight to that of the female tortoise fearful of being turned on her back during intercourse: She would likely be abandoned "to face the sky" after her partner is done with her (a highly unlikely situation in the reality of tortoise mating habits), thus "exposing her not only to the eagle (who is the devil) but also to the crows—the gossips, and slanderers who publicize her fault." Ferrand's treatise several times brings up the story of the virgins of Milesia as a cautionary tale. Inflamed by love, they ran wild in the marketplace and fell prey to suicidal urges. Nothing stopped this self-destructiveness until the authorities ordered that the bodies of those who had hanged themselves be cast out "naked on dung heaps." The prospect of sexual humiliation, even after death, was the best prophylactic.

Ironically, Ferrand also resorted to female shame as powerful medicine against *male* unrequited love. Under the watchful eye of the censorious ecclesiastic court of France, he parted ways from his "Mohammedan" predecessors who advised heartsick men to patronize prostitutes to evacuate *sperma*. A man who could not marry his conquest should take what writer Carol Neely calls the "misogyny cure." He should "meditate upon the imperfections and impurity of women." He must find a way to spy on her before she has brushed her hair and primped for the day. He might want to find a crone to egg him on; an old woman's withered limbs and wrinkled face would remind him of the inevitability of female ugliness in age. Ferrand related a particularly noxious trick of last resort: Hypatia, the brilliant daughter of Theon the geometrician and a mathematician in her own right, was so put off by the advances of one of her students that she reached under her skirt and pulled out a bloodied menstrual rag. "Look, young man," she cried. "You will see that what you love so much is nothing but vileness and filth." No matter which role a woman plays in unrequited love, she is the problem. Feeling impossible desire disgraces her, and so does being its object.

In the nineteenth century, romantic obsession took on a dual identity. It was seen as both a form of lovesickness and glorified as a spiritual and creative force. The French physician Jean-Étienne Esquirol saw romantic obsession as a form of monomania, a condition in which the sufferer focuses exhaustively and exclusively on one thing. Though monomania in a clinical context was considered a "partial insanity," it was also associated with art, learning, and great achievement. The expert with a single focus was a lauded figure, replacing the older ideal of the Renaissance man or woman who had a variety of skills and a wide breadth of knowledge. Professional specialists—doctors, composers, scientists, novelists—became more valued than generalists. The monomaniac, then, might end up in an asylum, or he might end up making a great discovery or creating a superlative work of art. The blurry distinction between the productive obsessive and the ruined one was an endless source of fascination in the Romantic era, played out most prominently in the character of Victor Frankenstein, the mad scientist obsessed with bringing life to the dead.

Obsessive love was its own kind of expertise, a quest to shape one's life entirely around a beloved. It offered the possibility of transformed consciousness and mystical oneness to the Romantics, who were intrigued by the altered mind-states that intense feeling, dreams, and madness could bring. The suffering that lovesickness entailed only gave it more credibility. Fictional female characters—chief among them Catherine in *Wuthering Heights*—swept up in this "partial insanity" fascinated readers. Lovesickness could be painfully glorious, a badge of honor rather than a label of shame.

Yet for the real women of the nineteenth century, the lovesickness diagnosis remained an oppressive one. The myth that women did not feel sexual desire still held sway in the public imagination. Women who were attracted to other women were unnatural "inverts." Women who were romantically obsessed, sexually voracious, or both were physical aberrations. One sure sign of a

woman's "amativeness," according to the emerging science of phre-
nology, was a larger than normal cerebellum, the area of the brain
located above the nape of the neck. Gynecologists believed uterine
disease (a catch-all phrase used to describe cramps, mood swings,
headaches, and other "disorders of the womb") caused erotomania,
Esquirol's term for fervent romantic obsession.

The labels, however, obscured what may have been a much
more important symptom: women's discontent with their limited
opportunities in love and life. Mary Sidgwick Benson was engaged
at twelve and married at eighteen to the man who would become
the archbishop of Canterbury. As she raised her infamously trying brood of children, she guiltily suffered unrequited longings,
which she called "swarmings," for other women. Later in her life,
she came to believe her feelings were not deviant urges but, rather,
"gifts from God" that she could and did act on. Her "lovesickness,"
then, drew her out of the heterosexual mandate and religious stric-
tures that stifled her. Lucy Tait, her female lover, eventually moved
in with the Benson family and became an accepted member of the
household. After the archbishop died in 1896, Tait took his place in
the marital bed.

Isabella Robinson's lovesickness did not have as happy an outcome. In one of the first cases heard under the 1857 law that made
divorce feasible for England's middle class, her husband, Henry,
sued her after he discovered her private diaries. The volumes described in detail her passion for Edward Lane, a young married
doctor and family friend, and several furtive intimate encounters
they had. Henry attempted to use the diaries to prove Isabella's infidelity; her attorneys argued that the entries were the result of de-
lusions caused by uterine disease, not evidence of an actual affair.
As Kate Summerscale details in *Mrs. Robinson's Disgrace: The
Private Diary of a Victorian Lady*, Isabella reluctantly accepted

the defense strategy because it was the only way she could save the career and reputation of her beloved Lane, who vehemently denied any indiscretion. Though she wanted to be rid of her husband, a divorce would turn her into an impoverished pariah, a fate she wanted to avoid.

For the many voyeuristic followers of the Robinson divorce case, the idea that Isabella was sick to the point of delusion offered a kind of solace as the institution of divorce unsettled British society. Women whose romantic obsessions took them, at least in their minds, outside the bonds of marriage were ill. Yet however much her unrequited love for Edward Lane made her suffer, Isabella privately insisted that the real problem was not medical. She was unhappy in her marriage but had no real options outside of it. She described her husband, a businessman who traveled frequently, as an "unpoetic soul" with a mean spirit. She was an intellectually curious and well-read woman who questioned religious authority and toyed with the then-radical ideas of atheism and evolutionism. She scribbled her illicit feelings for Dr. Lane in the pages of her diary, a volume meant to be private. But she also saw her passion as a force that exposed the limitations of her marriage. Lane, as she depicted him, cared deeply about her well-being, shared ideas with her, and listened attentively. In a different world, she would be free to pursue a better, more mutual relationship instead of being trapped in an oppressive marriage. In her diary, she pleaded for understanding from her imagined audience: "You see my inmost soul. You must despise and hate me," she wrote. "Do you also pause to pity?"

The medicalized Isabellas of the nineteenth century have since been overshadowed by the fictional heroines of romantic love, whose martyred longing represented an enviable emotional peak experience. *Wuthering Heights* has been remade into film no fewer than five times, *Jane Eyre* at least eighteen. The obsessive love narratives of romanticism, written with a level of detail that is itself obsessive, raised the bar on our expectations for love in the twentieth century, which were in turn amplified by the sexual revolution of the 1960s. Obsessive passion may be difficult and ultimately tragic, but its story is too compelling to be a mere cautionary tale. Romanticism presented a lasting emotional dare: How intense can you be? How powerfully can you love? Romantic obsession was no longer pathological. Love was *supposed* to consume and complete us. These ideas coincided with Western society's increasing skepticism about the existence of God and the reasons for ritual devotion. Love became our new religion, the target of our spiritual hunger, the place where we sought ecstasy, contentment, and awe. Obsessive love was as close as we could get to enlightenment, particularly as old mating systems—arranged marriages, formal dating rituals, rules of sexual conduct—fell away.

Psychologist Dorothy Tennov's 1979 bestseller *Love and Limerence* reflected these shifts. She criticized the psychologists and sociologists of her time for failing to fully acknowledge passionate love. The professional consensus then emphasized morality and rationality in love relationships; possessive, needy, unrequited, or irrational attachments were "masquerades," an immature state of dependency that was not really love. Tennov argued that passionate, obsessive love—what she called limerence—was a distinct yet common form of love, not an abnormality. She used written accounts and interviews with her research subjects, many of them her students at the University of Bridgeport, to demonstrate that the wild state the Romantic era so venerated was, for many people, a real phenomenon in relationships and crushes.

As I look back on how these ideas played out in my life before I got married, it all feels very twentieth-century. As a teenager and young adult in the 1980s and '90s, I fell in love a lot. The doped-up headiness of the experience *did* feel like a kind of transcendence. Any effort to stop myself from love, even when it was impractical or showed signs of being wrong for me, seemed like the denial of a fundamental right. When I wasn't in love, I was deeply lonely, beset by existential doubts: What if I never found love again? What if I died alone? So the motivation to seek love, however painful it might end up, usually outweighed the incentive to stay single. At times, though, I grew weary of taking all the bumps and pushed myself to be more independent. For a while I even tried to be more religiously observant, in part as an effort to find a surrogate for the faulty cycle of falling in and out of love.

As the century drew to a close, the era of romantic practicality was dawning. Obsessive unrequited love became not a grasping for transcendence but a sign of weakness. Women should stay cool and distant in the mating game. Romantic disappointment and obsessive love became problems women needed to stifle, as efficiently as possible, in the Machiavellian search for a mate. In 1998, the year of my obsession, I could have been a case study for everything a single woman was *not* supposed to do. My mate-finding strategy was focused on a man who wasn't available, yet I made myself available to him without conditions. I wasn't willing to get back in the game and consider other men. I was chasing much too hard. I was exactly the kind of woman the Dating Industrial Complex lampooned.

Around the same time, researchers began to gain unprecedented insight into the neurochemistry of love and attachment, and how pharmaceuticals might ease the impact of rejection. The idea of lovesickness gradually reemerged, with more empirical ammunition than ever before. Historically speaking, it hadn't been gone all that long.

❦

SAMARA, A THIRTY-TWO-YEAR-OLD legal assistant and writer, is in many ways a romantic. She is expert at the Old World art of letter writing and, for a time, ran a small business penning wedding vows and mash notes for others. The night before she moved to Philadelphia from New York City, she met Jim. They hit it off, and she bemoaned the fact that she'd come across such a great guy just as she was leaving town. He didn't seem to care that she would be living in another city. He wanted to see her again.

The weekends they spent together felt passionate and intimate. However, Samara soon realized Jim didn't mind the long-distance nature of their relationship because he had other women in his life. Yet the way he was when he was with her, she believed, suggested she was becoming more important to him. He took her to his office Christmas party and introduced her to his friends. She kept hoping he would choose to be with her exclusively. But he didn't.

Weeks would go by when she wouldn't hear from him. She grew increasingly preoccupied by these silences, scheming about when she might dare get in touch with him without seeming too intrusive. She spent a lot of time with her friends musing over his behavior. Once, after she told a friend how relieved she was to spend time with him after he'd been incommunicado for a while, the friend snapped at her: "You shouldn't see him anymore."

"But he apologized," Samara protested, and began to describe how tender their makeup had been.

"He apologized because he wanted to get laid," the friend said flatly.

Samara decided that she would keep quiet about the relationship. No matter how attentive Jim could be at times, he kept insisting he "didn't want a girlfriend." She didn't want her friends to know what she was putting up with. She was so caught up in what was increasingly becoming a one-sided relationship that she was unable to think of much else. Her mental state swung from one extreme to another. She fantasized about running into him at a moment when she was looking and feeling so great that he couldn't resist her. They'd start over and he would finally be hers. Then she would think about how much his behavior hurt her, and she would sink into a depression.

The situation became so distressing that Samara gathered the courage to cut off all communication. A few months later, she was in New York and ran into Jim at a Halloween party. He was with a woman dressed in a form-fitting Wonder Woman costume. She hated seeing him with someone else, but she consoled herself with the knowledge that he wasn't the commitment type. Wonder Woman was merely his latest conquest, and the couple would one day part ways, too. "I thought if I can't have him, no one can," Samara told me. "He was a fire that can't be contained."

Samara dated someone else for a while. After they broke up, her thoughts returned to Jim. She emailed him, thinking he might be up for one more whirlwind weekend together. He wrote back to decline. He and Wonder Woman were engaged.

Samara's story is something of a parable for every woman who ever believed her beloved is an incurable Lothario, or somehow psychologically broken, incapable of loving any woman in a lasting and real way. Such emotional cripples exist, but too often the reality is that he hasn't met his match yet, a woman whose powers of attraction seem, to the unwanted woman, nothing short of superheroic.

For Samara, the realization that she would never be that woman magnified and darkened her obsession with Jim. She was so distraught that she woke up every morning with dry heaves and felt a pressure "like a hippopotamus on my chest." She could not stop crying. She couldn't eat or work. She didn't understand why her reaction was so extreme, far beyond what she would consider a normal response to unrequited love. She had a happy childhood. She is very close to her family, particularly her father, whom she describes as steady and committed, "the opposite" of Jim. The only thing that seemed to be wrong with her was that her heart was broken, and it was taking over her life. "I was so embarrassed," she said.

She went to a therapist, who told her she likely had a disorder she'd never heard of: limerence. Whereas Dorothy Tennov used the term in the 1970s to describe what she saw as the normal, though difficult, condition of being in passionate love, Samara's therapist used it in a distinctly different way. Limerence still meant the involuntary state of being in love and experiencing an overwhelming and preoccupying need to have those feelings returned. But it was no longer considered a "normal human experience" in the way Tennov described it. Instead, limerence described a disorder.

This new view of limerence evolved after Tennov's death in 2007. Albert Wakin, a psychology professor at Sacred Heart University in Fairfield, Connecticut, and a former colleague of Tennov, was granted access to her archives, which were so prodigious that they filed an entire room in her son's house. What struck Wakin as he sorted through the boxes and files were the letters Tennov had received from readers after the publication of *Love and Limerence*. Many of them detailed stories of enduring and painful obsession. One woman bemoaned the fact that she was fixated on a boyfriend who'd left her ten years before. Another knew she should be happy in her life as a wife and mother, but her life was clouded by persistent thoughts of a man she'd met before her marriage. These situations, Wakin realized, were not romantic and not normal. "These were problem relationships," he told me.

Wakin has since reconceptualized limerence as pathology, fitting to the era of romantic practicality. It's often hard to recognize the problem, since limerence and the ardent feeling of new love are a lot alike. You can't stop thinking about the beloved. You're euphoric yet insecure, always in need of his attention. Your energy is up. Yet while new love settles down after six to twenty-four months into a calmer, more contented mutual relationship, people with limerence are stuck in this state of *amour fou*, which persists no matter whether the relationship breaks up or never forms at all. Limerence can plague even a relationship that lasts, when one or both partners are perpetually needy, obsessed, and insecure about the partnership—a condition also known as "relationship obsessive-compulsive disorder."

Wakin says limerence has features of both OCD and substance addiction. Addicts need more and more of their drug of preference to get high and spend more and more of their time getting it. People with limerence are never satisfied with the attention they get; if they're not getting any, they can't stop themselves from seeking it. Both addicts and people with limerence suffer physically and emotionally if they can't get their fix, and both struggle to kick the habit—or know they should. OCD sufferers live in a state of anxiety and obsession, which is reduced temporarily only by performing a certain behavior—hand washing, for example, to allay invasive worries about germs and disease. The obsessed lover's worries, in turn, may be briefly assuaged by signs of reassurance, real or imagined, from the beloved, but then the anxiety builds anew. Yet limerence is more than a hybrid of addiction and OCD. The interpersonal factors—what happens between the obsessed lover and the object of her desire—can make limerence more extreme and more complex. "Limerence can likely become the strongest kind of OCD and addiction that can be felt," Wakin told me. "Although alcohol and gambling can consume you, casinos and liquor don't have a life of their own. They don't remind you that they are still alive. They don't make you wonder what they're doing when they're not paying attention to you. So when you're obsessed with another living person, the obsession is even stronger."

Wakin would like to see limerence become an entry in the *Diagnostic and Statistical Manual of Mental Disorders* (DSM), the professional bible used by clinicians and psychiatrists to diagnose psychiatric illnesses (and by insurance companies as a basis for claims coding). The process of getting something new into the *DSM* is long and complicated, and Wakin is just getting started on building a body of research. But his nascent mission has gone quietly viral among brokenhearted Web surfers and has attracted considerable media attention. Every time his work is mentioned in the media, he fields a fresh onslaught of emails and calls from people who tell him that reading about his research gave them a shock of recognition.

Wakin's work is an outgrowth of mounting scientific evidence of the similarities among love, addiction, and OCD. Helen Fisher, a biological anthropologist who studies romantic love, says that "romantic love is an addiction: a perfectly wonderful addiction when it's going well, and a perfectly horrible addiction when it's going poorly." Fisher and her colleagues have used functional magnetic resonance imaging (fMRI) to see how blood flows through the brain of people who are passionately in love and people who've been rejected by someone they're still in love with. When the subjects looked at photographs of their beloved, one of the areas where blood flow increased was the ventral tegmental area (VTA), causing it to glow on the fMRI scan—an indication that a region of the brain is becoming more active. Located in the "reptilian core" of the brain, the VTA generates the neurotransmitter dopamine, a natural stimulant that gives you energy, focus, feelings of euphoria, and, most important, that yen to seek out a particular beloved. The VTA also becomes active when people use cocaine—an indication that the expression "lover's high" is grounded in a very real physical phenomenon.

So when you're in passionate love, whether reciprocated or not, you truly are in a state of craving. What makes matters more intense is that being in love causes a decline in the levels of another neurotransmitter, serotonin, which is involved in regulating aggression, mood, and anxiety. A study by the Italian psychiatrist Donatella Marazziti uncovered a striking similarity between people with OCD and people in love. Both groups had serotonin levels 40 percent lower than the control group. While couples in the tumult of romance can find refuge in the soothing effects of oxytocin—the so called "cuddle chemical"—and vasopressin—believed to foster attachment—the unrequited lover can't catch a break from anxious obsession.

What all this means, according to Fisher and her research team, is that passionate love is fundamentally a drive meant to propel us toward the reward of attachment with a specific mate. When we're deprived of that reward, our neurochemistry keeps pushing us to get it back in a phenomenon known as "frustration attraction." After romantic rejection, blood flow increases not only to the VTA, but also to brain areas related to deep emotional attachment, addictive behavior, and physical pain. We become even more enamored. Our longing for contact worsens. We literally hurt. And we try to figure out what happened. Areas of the forebrain region, associated with responding to gains and losses, lit up on the fMRI scans. This suggests that bereft lovers mull over how the rejection occurred and what they can do to get back the rejecter, the source of the love fix.

OBSESSIVE LOVE'S KINSHIP with addiction and OCD influences how we perceive human passion. There's nothing transcendent about a system neurochemically out of wack. Science journalism in the era of romantic practicality regularly feasts on stories about the boom-and-bust neurology of love, with headlines such as "New Love: A Short Shelf Life" and "Anti-Love Drug May Be Ticket to Bliss." We need to love more sanely, argues psychiatrist Frank Tallis, and not overvalue passion and romance. He's one of the many thinkers who extol the satisfaction rates among couples in arranged marriages, which rival or exceed those of couples in marriages of choice—the takeaway message being that our own faulty hearts aren't very good guides to marital success. In her book *Marry Him!*, Lori Gottlieb advises women not to hold out for Mr. Right and instead seek out "Mr. Good Enough." She questions the notion that you need "great chemistry" for real love to develop. Chemistry, she points out, causes you to ignore work, compulsively check your email, and act foolishly—and often doesn't lead to anything lasting. Susan Cheever, who wrote a book exploring her long-term misguided obsession with a hard-drinking journalist, admonishes the tendency to reflexively celebrate love under any circumstances. Why should our friends and family be happy for us to be obsessed with a person when they would be horrified if we were so enslaved to gin, meth, or overeating?

When obsession besets the unrequited lover, it seems even more pathological. The unwanted woman is running on empty, with no substantial evidence that her love is going anywhere. Wakin told me that it's usually not appropriate to diagnose limerence until the relationship in question has lasted at least six months, the point when heady preoccupation begins to give way to a more predictable and stable connection. "But sometimes I have someone tell me, 'I've met someone and I'm on an emotional roller coaster and they hardly know I exist'—and we can look at that as a problem from the beginning," he said.

When I first began to understand the neurochemistry of passionate love, I took great comfort in the idea that what had happened to me might be a distinct disorder with a scientific explanation. I *had* felt addicted and out of control. Throughout my twenties, I suffered bouts of clinical depression, several of them related to the end of a relationship. Had I reached for B., then, like a junkie going for her fix? The science seemed fairly neutral, not a tool of oppression, like older ideas of lovesickness. And the emergence of the limerence as a diagnosis is accompanied by the possibility of more promising cures. Wakin advises obsessed lovers to pursue cognitive behavioral therapy, a treatment that helps them change their perceptions about their beloved. Antidepressants, he tells them, can be an effective approach as well. Samara, who contacted Wakin at the suggestion of her therapist, started taking a low dose of the antidepressant Lexapro, which, along with therapy, helped her move on. She still thought of Jim, but by the time he walked down the aisle with Wonder Woman, Samara was no longer obsessed. She could compartmentalize her feelings enough to concentrate at work and go out with friends. She presented her story as one of empowerment through diagnosis and treatment, a significant contrast to the historical examples I've related.

Using an elixir to blunt the power of obsessive love seems somehow inevitable. If we're turning increasingly to Ambien to help us sleep, Adderall to help us concentrate, and Wellbutrin to ward off anxiety and depression, why not a pill for off-the-rails desire? Advances in neuroscience and pharmacology seem very likely to lead to a variety of "chemical breakup" remedies to treat problematic passions. Although I don't question Samara's decision to turn to therapy and medication, the comfort I took in her story of over-coming limerence was shadowed by the issues that arise with our contemporary pharmaceutical toolbox and the mounting number of diagnoses that justify our reliance on it. We medicate jumpy children so they can endure elementary school classrooms that require them to sit still for most of the day. Leaders of an Israeli ultra-Orthodox Jewish community compel psychiatrists to pre-scribe medication to help teens and married couples comply with strict rules on masturbation and sexual intercourse. And some sec-ular folk admit to taking antidepressants in order to endure their spouses and preserve their marriages.

The issue is more intricate than that, of course. Plenty of parents testify that the right attention-calibrating drugs have saved their children from serious behavior and learning problems. Chronic de-pression that goes untreated is ruinous, whether it besets a spouse or someone dealing with the blow of rejection. And romantic ob-session and stalking can be features of serious, less common psychi-atric disorders that need medical attention: borderline personality disorder, psychopathy, and erotomania, whose sufferers are under the delusion that someone else, usually of a higher social status, is in love with them.

But as lovesickness reemerges as a diagnosis with a potentially vast applicability, we need to ask the same question prompted by other increasingly widespread disorders. The meds may help ease the devastating pain of rejection in situations when the anguish doesn't seem to cease. Yet serotonin-regulating drugs also may di-minish people's ability to feel deep human attachment and sexual desire, forces that spur reproduction and make the human expe-rience richer, albeit more challenging and complex. If the use of these pharmaceuticals is too vast and too indiscriminate, we risk zombifying our love life, if we bother to have one.

Medication obscures another key question behind the strife of unrequited love: Is the problem just with the patient, or is it also in the conditions of her life?

Samara told me that after she felt better, she started going out with an attorney. They had a great first date and dated a lot over the next two months. When an essay she wrote about her limerence diagnosis was published in a popular women's magazine, she felt confident enough with him to tell him about it. When he stopped calling not long after, she had no idea whether the article had scared him away or if he'd been put off by a recent weekend trip that hadn't gone as well as she'd expected. She was disappointed but not distraught. She had been careful, she told me, not to "give myself to him," as she felt she'd done with Jim. She had no regrets. It was part of who she was to write openly about her life. She sounded wise and cautious, enviably self-possessed.

But her story is shadowed by that nagging doubt: Did her brave and public confession of her distress undermine her in the new guy's mind, even though she'd clearly bounced back? Did her story suggest to him that at some point she might be more fragile, more high-maintenance? Or was he just feeling like it was time to move on? The no-guarantees attitude of romance today has its own way of being oppressive, permitting lovers a mincing fickleness. The cost-benefit analysis relationship formation has become an extreme sport. As one of the female characters in Adelle Waldman's novel, *The Love Affairs of Nathaniel P.*, puts it, "Dating is probably the most fraught human interaction there is. You're sizing people up to see if they're worth your time and attention, and they're doing the same to you. It's a meritocracy applied to personal life, but there's no accountability." Lexapro and therapy helped prevent Samara from taking disappointment too much to heart. Perhaps these remedies serve another purpose: to make the unwanted woman a more resilient, lower-maintenance, less-likely-to-put-up-a-fuss citizen of the Dating Industrial Complex. Maybe this is the new "place" that women, with their independence and economic self-sufficiency in a world of romantic uncertainty, are supposed to occupy.

ANTIDEPRESSANTS DIDN'T PREVENT Alice, a thirty-nine-year-old woman in Southern California, from becoming romantically obsessed. She's been on SSRIs for years, part of a regimen for treating her bipolar disorder. She gave up her profession as a university administrator because the waves of mania and depression made it difficult for her to hold down a job. She spent most of her time alone. Her husband, a corporate executive, worked long days, then went to the gym for a couple of hours, intent on maintaining his weight loss. When Alice eloped with him when they were in college, he weighed three hundred pounds and had been fat since childhood. His size didn't matter to her. He was a stable, loving force in her life, someone who helped her flee the chaos of her teens. Her father was out of work and she had been expected to help care for her five younger siblings. She acted out instead, causing so much trouble that she was kicked out of two different schools.

Alice and her husband had a good sex life at first. But as her bipolar disorder worsened and he lost weight, he became less interested in making love to her. He was critical of her body— she'd put on some weight because her medication slowed down her thyroid—and he was preoccupied with maintaining his own. "Losing weight changed him a lot," Alice said. "Whatever that took mentally is affecting whatever it takes to let go and have sex. He was more sensual and free when he was fat."

He was also intensely protective of her. He came to seem more like a parent than a spouse. When I interviewed Alice, she told me he hadn't kissed her deeply in ten years. "He's just into this thing where he's my guardian," she said. "He calls me 'little girl.' He buys me whimsical presents."

A year after Alice stopped working, she told her husband that she wanted to take classes at the local community college. He agreed but insisted that she enroll in only one course at a time. She chose a basic drawing class. Slater, the teacher, was an artist her own age. The first week, he gave her a big smile when it was her turn to introduce herself. "It was like a lightning bolt," she said. "I never knew that even existed, the love-at-first-sight kind of thing."

Thus began what Alice described as an intensely sexual flirtation. She baked banana bread and cookies for Slater. After she told him she liked the David Bowie song he'd played during class, Slater played more of Bowie's music. He brushed up against her when he was looking at her drawings. A group of students in the class moved their desks to get a better view of the flirtation. Every class, there were lots of "tiny subtle things" that passed between them. He teased her a lot, and she welcomed his playfulness; her husband was introverted and more serious. Alice knew Slater was also married, and she told herself that perhaps he saw her as a safe way to express himself sexually without consequences.

Her feelings built. She sought him out online. She went to ratemyprofessors.com and gave him a rave review with a red chili pepper—a sign that a student finds a professor intellectually-slash-sexually "hot." She went on an art website where he kept a page of his work and commented extensively on it. She used a pseudonym, then alluded to things she'd done or said in class to let on who she really was. He responded, thanking her avatar and complimenting her for her ability to write about art.

Her thoughts were most intense at night, after she shut down her laptop and got into bed with her husband, who insisted that she end her day when he did. "He feels he has to watch over me," she said. "He's scared of the bipolar, and he tries to control me. We joke that I'm this rag doll he takes to bed with him." After her husband fell asleep, Alice would lie awake and think of Slater. She composed letters to him in her head. Her flirtation, though it remained platonic, felt like her only sex life, she told me more than once during our conversation. "It was this whole sexual intellectual high," she said. "I hadn't interacted like that for a long time. It was exhilarating and intense."

After the semester ended, Alice went to an opening of a show of Slater's work. She lied to her husband about where she was going. At the show, Slater asked her to take his class the following semester. The way he asked felt sweet and romantic to Alice. When she got into bed with her husband that night, she burst into tears. She confessed that she'd lied about where she had been. Then she told him the more important truth: She was in love with her art teacher.

Her husband was furious. He told her he wanted a divorce. The prospect that their marriage might be ending threw Alice into confusion. She had dreamed of living on her own. She had mused that maybe one day Slater would leave his wife to be with her. But she was terrified of being without her husband. She called Slater and pleaded with him to make her stop feeling what she was feeling. "Block me from your email, block me from your number," she begged. Slater protested that he didn't know how to do that—and insisted there was nothing to stop. He was just being friendly, he explained. "I'm committed to my wife," he said.

Alice and her husband didn't break up. The threat of divorce sent her spiraling into depression. Her husband was there to take care of her, just as he always had been. She didn't sign up for another class with Slater.

At times Alice sees her obsession with Slater as pure chemistry, lovesickness linked to her bipolar disorder. Her feelings were "part of a rising hypomania," a high-energy state that drove her to write the long commentaries online about his art and to believe that his feelings were equally avid. In reality, she barely knew him. "He's an outline of a human man, and it's static inside," she said.

But her romantic obsession, like Isabella Robinson's, allowed her to look beyond the confines of the circumscribed life she and her husband had created to protect her from stress and keep her bipolar condition under control. Her feelings about Slater, she told me, were a projection of a part of herself. "He's an artist," she told me. "I'm jealous of him. I didn't make a good career choice when I was younger. I can't work a nine-to-five job. I need to do something with my hands, something I can do alone. He's doing something I wish I had done."

She related her infatuation to the Jungian notion of the anima and the animus, the respective feminine and masculine aspects of our collective unconscious. Men tend to repress the anima, the emotional, receptive, sensitive, caretaking feminine side. Women will do the same to the animus, which represents physical power, creative accomplishment, action, public expression, and the search for meaning.

Jung's wife and colleague, Emma Jung, helped develop these ideas. Her two classic papers, published together as *Animus and Anima* in 1957, detail a phenomenon very much like the romantic obsession Alice described. A woman projects the animus onto a man she loves because her masculine side feels dangerous to her. Projection is a defense, a way of not owning her feelings and experiences. But the projection can also create a "compulsive tie," as it did to Alice—what Emma Jung described as a "dependence on him that often increases to the point of being unbearable." She urged people to recognize the projection and dismantle it. Only then can they get in touch with their masculine side and harness it to guide them to their own power. "We're always looking for that missing piece in ourselves," said Jungian analyst Jacqueline Wright. "That ideal lover or person that we're looking for holds a quality that we don't recognize or express in ourselves."

This theory is one possible interpretation of what was happening to Alice, with no hard science behind it. But the idea resonated strongly for her. Powerful aspects of her self—her rebelliousness, her sexuality, her need to create and have purpose in her life—had been tamped down to keep her mental illness in check. There certainly was reason for caution. Her illness has caused her and her husband great pain. At times she has been suicidal. But the depth of her obsession raised questions about whether the tight restrictions on her life might have backfired in sexual, emotional, and creative frustration. Alice wasn't really obsessed with Slater. She was obsessed with what was missing in her life. The real romantic possibility here—of a more fulfilled existence—was one that might very well be within reach.

In our time, seeing romantic obsession mainly as pathology closes a window in our psyches. The label of "sick" as opposed to "healthy" in love is often code for what's inconvenient, messy, annoying, and confusing. In our eagerness to categorize yearning, we may neglect to ask what we are truly yearning for. If we dismiss romantic obsession as nothing more than a tumor to be excised from our psyche, we'll see no reason to heed what our longing might be trying to tell us.

4

Boy Chasers

THE (FE)MALE URGE TO PURSUE

ᴡ

BEFORE I BECAME OBSESSED WITH B.,
he told me about a new staging of *A Streetcar Named Desire* that was all the rage among
theater scholars. Stanley was played by a
woman, Blanche by a man. I laughed. "Sounds
liberating."

The idea quickly caught on between us.
The first time I invited him out for a drink,
his emailed response read: *Dear Stanley: Yes,
I would like very much to have a beer. What
night is good for you? Blanche DuBois.* I replied: *Dear Blanche: Maybe after my Monday
night class? I'm free at 8:30. Stanley.*

The exchange seemed like more than a flirtatious joke. I had been spending a lot of time

at the gym that summer, lifting weights to fight my sadness over the end of my relationship. The amount I could lift, push, and pull was gradually increasing. I felt my strength at other times, too, opening the heavy stairwell doors at school, or carrying my bicycle up and down my apartment stairs. Whenever I made a fist and bent my elbow, the new muscle rising from my forearm seemed like someone else's. I was the kind of girl who was picked last for teams in gym class in elementary school. I'd never tried to be strong before. Had B. noticed I looked different? I let myself feel flattered.

As for Blanche, B. was tall and thin, with a sharp nose, a repertoire of expressive hand gestures, and an air of being too intelligent to stay in the confines of one gender. What was evolving between us felt new—a relationship in which gender roles were playful choices, not dictates. I had never bought into the idea that the man was supposed to make the first moves and the woman was supposed to play it cool. That game seemed retrograde and dishonest, though it was always *there* somehow: If I wait until he kisses me first, I'm behaving. If I go ahead and do it, I am transgressing— but that wasn't a bad thing. In fact, it could carry a certain erotic charge, with the message: *I want you enough to break the rules.*

As my obsession with B. took hold, the role reversal intensified. I became the steadfast knight, shadowing him unseen, waiting and planning for the moments when I might get a dose of his attention. He played the girlie game of keeping me guessing and yearning. He wavered between devotion to his out-of-town girlfriend and what seemed like a clear attraction to me. He would confess he wanted me back, then ward me off by saying he needed more time.

A couple of times we ended up in each other's arms. As we kissed and touched, I'd have the sense of a clock ticking loudly somewhere, counting off the moments before an alarm would go off in his tortured conscience, making him stop. We kept up the gender-bending banter. One night after he stopped me from taking off his pants, he joked, "Sorry to be such a cock tease."

The line unsettled me because it felt so appropriate. All the ways male desire had ever been described to me—its mind-consuming, nearly painful *insistence*—seemed to be my new reality. I felt like I really *was* becoming Stanley, standing on a fire escape in a white T-shirt, bellowing my beloved's name without caring what the neighbors thought.

THERE MAY HAVE been a neurobiological basis for what I was feeling. Research indicates that men and women go through similar neurochemical and hormonal changes when they fall in love, with one interesting distinction: Testosterone, the hormone associated with sex drive and aggression, goes up in women and decreases in men. How this testosterone fluctuation affects our behavior hasn't been studied yet. But University of Pisa neuroscientist Donatella Marazziti, who led the testosterone research, surmised that the changes in female and male body chemistry may be meant to bring the sexes closer together in love—"as if nature wants to eliminate what can be different in men and women."

Women do, then, become hormonally more "masculine" when they're love-struck. Confessed one woman I interviewed, who hadn't known about Marazziti's findings, "I just *felt* like I had more testosterone. I felt more stringy and muscular. It was totally bizarre." The testosterone increase is accompanied by a rise in cortisol (which occurs in both sexes), a hormone associated with stress and physiological arousal—our fight-or-flight response. The more thinking you tend to do about the relationship, one study found, the more cortisol levels increase. In a reciprocated relationship, the cortisol rise happens along with stress-*reducing* responses: an increase in positive emotions and the release of oxytocin and vasopressin. The unrequited lover, in contrast, is stuck in thought, with fewer—if any—of these calming forces, her body hormonally primed to take action.

This hormonal shift is one of many factors that indicate a more complex reality behind the long-standing ideal that women are supposed to be the pursued in love, not the pursuers. Historically, our culture has coped with this reality by tagging lustful boy chasers as women who aren't fully female. Hippocrates cautioned that longing and sexual frustration could literally transform a woman into a man; he believed that the heat of desire could reverse female genitals and turn them into penises, a superstition that endured through the Renaissance. Desire—along with the freedom to travel alone, carry weapons, have adventures, and enjoy a host of other privileges—belonged to men. If women wanted any of these privileges, they needed not so much a set of male genitals as a set of male clothes. In masculine garb, some daring women got away with venturing unescorted into the world. Shakespeare linked this freedom with the freedom to pursue love, as cross-dressing gave *Twelfth Night*'s Viola and several other Shakespearean heroines cover and authority to successfully win over their love interests.

In Victor Hugo's *Les Misérables*, wearing men's clothes allowed the street urchin Éponine to join her beloved, Marius, at the barricades, where she took a fatal bullet for him. Éponine's cross-dressing foreshadowed the real-life masculine disguises donned by Hugo's own daughter Adèle as she sought out the object of her obsession, the British soldier Albert Pinson. Perhaps she purposely copied the tactics of Éponine, who, unlike the character in the Broadway musical, was portrayed as unseemly and conniving until her redemptive self-sacrifice for Marius, a student revolutionary. Adèle's obsession started when she was twenty-six and propelled her to follow Pinson to Halifax and then Barbados. At age forty-one, she returned to her parents, her expression blank and her conversation limited to exchanges with the voices in her head. Hugo placed her in an expensive asylum outside of Paris, where she would live for the rest of her life. He visited Adèle in the company of his longtime mistress, whose own daughter was buried nearby. "We went together to Saint-Mandé," Hugo wrote. "She goes to see her daughter in the cemetery, alas!, and I go to see mine."

It's crucial to consider Adèle's life before her obsession took hold. As a young woman, she was beautiful and intense. She chafed at the protectiveness of her father, who was known to the world as a model parent, yet at home maintained an unbending authority. She was musically gifted. She performed her piano compositions in public to some acclaim, and a visiting composer urged her to publish her music. Hugo derided his daughter's talent and considered her playing a distraction to his work. He didn't want her to do much else, either. He protested his wife's efforts to take Adèle on a trip abroad so she could get away from the boredom of life in Guernsey, the remote British island where the family lived in exile from the time she was a teenager. He also despised Adèle's idol, the feminist writer George Sand. Hugo called Sand "a dangerous model" and disdained her ideas about equal rights for women.

Yet Adèle was greatly influenced by Sand's writings, in particular her arguments against marriage. When, early in their courtship, Pinson asked Adèle to marry him, she turned him down, as she'd done with four other suitors. Then she changed her mind. She tried to get Pinson back, only to discover that his affections had waned. Her unrequited love for him would define the rest of her life. In the pages of her diary, she expressed her love in terms that reflected the self-absorbed privilege of unilateral desire: her effort to assert her selfhood through the idea of her beloved. "You are . . . a man of the past who loves a woman of the future," she wrote. "I love you as the sculptor loves the clay." After he was transferred to Halifax, she hatched a plan to follow him there, a bold move for a single woman, even at thirty-two. She had a lot at stake. Her pursuit of Pinson was about much more than winning his love; it was about escaping her father's grip and seizing control over her own destiny. She wrote of her intentions in her diary:

> *It would be an incredible thing if a young woman,*
> *who is so enslaved that she cannot even go out to buy*
> *paper, went to sea and sailed from the Old World to the*
> *New to be with her love. This thing I shall do.*
> *It would be an incredible thing if a young woman,*
> *whose only sustenance is the crust of bread her father*
> *deigns to give her, had in her possession, four years*
> *from now, money earned by honest toil, money of her*
> *own. This thing I shall do.*

Adèle's goal of remaking herself on her own terms became enmeshed with her desire to win a man who no longer cared for her. She made the voyage to Halifax, where Pinson was stationed, and pursued him there for the next six years. Her landlady wrote to her brother that she often went out at night dressed in men's evening wear, searching for Pinson. Though Éponine may have been on her mind, Adèle likely took her cues from Sand, whose male pseudonym and attire helped her access male privilege; she could move about Paris more freely and enter places otherwise forbidden to women. For Adèle to go after what she wanted in life and in love demanded a manly guise that would allow her to venture out into the dark streets to try to win back her beloved. This costume, so integral to her tragic story, was immortalized by François Truffaut, who included a scene of Adèle, played by the young Isabelle Adjani, in a black top hat and suit in his 1975 film based on Adèle's life, *L'Histoire d'Adèle H.*

IN MOST OF the Western world today, women don't need male clothing to travel unescorted, and they earn their money by "honest toil" alongside men. Yet our culture still sees as not quite female the woman who takes the initiative in the quest for love. She's somehow manly, a behavioral cross-dresser, like the horny she-to-he of Hippocrates's imagination. And like Adèle Hugo, she's doomed to fail. In psychologist Tracy McMillan's 2012 best seller *Why You're Not Married . . . Yet: The Straight Talk You Need to Get the Relationship You Deserve,* reason #9 (after #7, "You Hate Yourself," and #8, "You're a Liar") is "You're a Dude." She advises women to stop thinking that women's equality means they can act like men in the dating game. Her cautionary tale is a woman named Valerie, who is "too deep in her Masculine" and fools herself by thinking that "women fought for the right to be equal, and that means acting just like men in every area of life." Valerie dares to strike up conversations with men, call and text them, and ask for dates. "After a decade of dating 'equally' she is in a long-term relationship with exactly *none* of the men she has pursued!" McMillan gloats.

I can't weigh in on whether McMillan is right. This isn't a book of dating advice. Though if you've ever sat around and talked with long-term couples about how their relationships started, you'll likely find plenty that didn't follow the "let the guy be the pursuer" formula. Finding mutual love often works very differently from the unilateral pursue-and-persuade mission that men are supposedly programmed to conduct. It's more likely to be a gradual exchange and interpretation of signals of interest, part of the "reconnaissance dance" of figuring out if you want to be together.

Anyone, female or male, who comes on too strong risks turning off the other person and being perceived as needy or aggressive—but the pop-psychology cautionary tales for these "high-maintenance" types almost invariably have a female protagonist.

All Valerie seems like is a gal who doesn't hesitate to make the first move, not a desperate stalker. And she isn't alone. Straight women say they initiate about 40 percent of their relationships. When you break down courtship into distinct behaviors, the research shows that men and women pursue relationships at similar rates and act in similar ways. A 2005 study of undergraduates at the University of Pittsburgh reveals that almost all women and men use what psychologists call repeated "approach behaviors"— sending messages, doing favors, starting conversations, asking for dates—when they're trying to get someone interested in them or trying to win back a partner after a relationship ends. Most men and women engage in what the study calls "surveillance": They hang out in places where their beloveds are likely to be, pass by their homes, join the same activities, and try to tease information out of mutual friends about their prospects of success.

"There are expectations that women are the passive recipients of male courtship behaviors," said Stacey L. Williams, a psychology professor at East Tennessee State University and the lead author of the study. "Our societal expectations and norms in that way are not really true. The stereotypes don't hold up."

Three additional large-scale studies on how people react to rejection confirm that women engage in pursuit behaviors at similar rates to men. The range of behaviors studied—from asking someone out to harassment—means that these findings are not necessarily cause for celebration. The question of when pursuit goes overboard is a critical one and a central concern of this book, but I'll set the issue aside for a moment to underscore the basic disparity revealed by these studies: The ideal of the male pursuer/female pursued is very, very far from reality.

Why, then, does the courtship double standard have so much staying power? The notion that men are the natural chasers in the mating game is rooted in the "parental investment theory" of evolutionary psychology. Because of their biology, men and women put vastly different levels of investment into perpetuating their genes. Men don't have to spend much time and energy on reproduction. But they do have to compete for a scarcer pool of female mates—scarcer not because there are fewer females but because women are available for reproduction less often than men. Women can add to the species only one long pregnancy at a time, while men can "spread their seed" with far greater frequency. That makes men the pursuers, hardwired to court and chase. By extension, women are the choosers, evaluating mate prospects on the basis of the resources they might provide to them and their offspring. A woman needs to assess whether a man will stick around to make sure she and their spawn will have food, shelter, and other resources during the high-need times of pregnancy, birth, infancy, and early childhood.

This baseline theory is reiterated in various watered-down forms in the rhetoric of the Dating Industrial Complex. A woman is supposed to play the chooser by refraining from taking the initiative in romance, thus providing the impression that she is of "high value" or a "prize," while a man thrives on competition and "the thrill of the chase." These tactics, which advise an almost Victorian-era level of self-control (relationship expert Matthew Hussey goes so far as to advocate for a modern version of the "white handkerchief approach"—the hanky-dropping tactic Victorian women used to let a man know of her interest), may certainly be useful. Men are authorized to go after what they want. Even if they have to submit to the boss lady at work, at the bar they can play the ego-gratifying roles of the bold hunter or calculating "pickup artist." The anesthetized narratives of advice books portray both genders in a winning light, if they follow the protocol: The boy gets to "get" the girl. The girl is encouraged to feel like the one who's in control all along by being quietly confident in her passive Feminine self. Whether this pose gives her genuine power, though, is called into question by the experiences of women such as Maria, who followed her mother's advice to "let them come to you"—and ended up feeling that she had no real choice in her life partner.

When the male pursuer/female pursued model is effective, it's not because the roles bring us back to our essential male and female mating selves. In the animal world, females in a number of mammal species are the mating pursuers. This is the case with rats and several primate species: orangutans, bonobos, and several kinds of monkeys, including rhesus monkeys, which are genetically so close to us that they served as stand-ins to see if humans could survive trips to the moon. As journalist Daniel Bergner points out in *What Do Women Want?: Adventures in the Science of Female Desire*, these creatures don't contend with any cultural messages about how the sexes should and shouldn't behave—which raises the question of whether the "male pursuer" mandate is biologically or socially constructed.

Even evolutionary psychology allows that gender roles in mating are flexible, meant to respond to stress and change, to ecological and biological realities. Glenn Geher, my colleague at the State University of New York at New Paltz, is an evolutionary psychology professor and the co-author of *Mating Intelligence Unleashed: The Role of the Mind in Sex, Dating, and Love*. He explained that the female urge to pursue is more likely to kick in when the reproductive tables are turned. Her position as chooser weakens as she ages and her fertility declines—the so-called cougar phenomenon. "There's probably a tipping point when females stop having an upper hand in mating," he said. Correspondingly, even fertile younger women may be more likely to chase in situations where there aren't many men. Both scenarios—women looking for mates later in their reproductive lives and majority-female environments—are increasingly common, particularly for educated women and men. The average age of a first-time mother is rising. Women outnumber men on college campuses nationwide.

Taking into account environmental and situational variables, then, romantic pursuit becomes less about what men and women fundamentally are (or should be) and more about a way of responding to a real or perceived condition of mate scarcity. It seems no coincidence that for college women, becoming more professionally successful is also connected to diminished mating prospects; enhancing your own ability to provide is another way of taking charge when the competition for mates and their resources goes up. Yet while we've come to accept female determination in the work world, female perseverance still rankles in matters of love.

NO MATTER WHAT the environmental factors are, the proclivity to get hung up on a particular someone is vital to the survival of our species. Romantic obsession and pursuit are adaptations for both men and women in the mating game. We focus exclusively on one person because it fosters pair bonds, which help us raise offspring successfully. "It takes a long time to go through a pregnancy and take care of a child," said social psychologist Arthur Aron. "Having both parents helps the child survive. If our ancestors didn't have a strong motivation to bond and connect, we might not be here as a species." So what drives us to jealousy and pursuit is integrally linked to the forces that create us and make us thrive, even though, like many fundamental human motivations, the drive to bond, as Aron put it, "can run awry."

ANGELA, A TRANSLATOR in her mid-forties, met Heinrich at a run-down hostel in Augsburg while she was spending a year teaching in Germany. She was twenty-five, and he was about to turn thirty. "He had these piercing blue eyes," she said. "I remember not being able to look at him because his gaze was so bright."

Heinrich made it clear he wanted to see her again. He gave her his address in former East Berlin, an exotic place to her in the wake of the fall of the Berlin Wall, and he encouraged her to visit. A couple of months later, she traveled to the city with a friend. They didn't know anyone there, so they bought a bottle of wine and stopped by Heinrich's apartment unannounced. The three spent the evening drinking together. He invited Angela to return.

It was a time in her life when she felt "extremely unmoored." Her adolescence and early twenties had been consumed by a relationship with a much older man. Her job in Germany was giving her some badly needed confidence. But she also felt alone. "All of a sudden I was out there in the world trying to figure things out on my own," she said. "I hadn't ever learned to be a grown up by myself. I wasn't used to feeling like an adult without a man to guide me."

The next time she was in Berlin, she met Heinrich for drinks. He kissed her. His assertiveness "marked him as a good beacon" for her, she remembered—he was what she thought she needed to feel more settled. And then she was smitten.

Heinrich visited her in Stuttgart, where she was teaching. They fell into bed. She was astonished when he entered her without using a condom. They hadn't talked about whether she was on birth control. Before the next time they made love, she bought condoms and gave them to him. He didn't use them, though, so she started taking birth control pills.

Their affair lasted just a few weeks. When she came to see him, he would greet her at the train with two bicycles. "East Berlin was all about bicycling, so I was riding around on my perfect Eastern bicycle. It was great," she said. "I dreamed what was happening into this fantasy, and he was providing the props for me to live it out."

She arrived one weekend on the eve of his thirtieth birthday. They planned to celebrate the next day with his friends. Soon after she got to his apartment, he excused himself to make a phone call. There was no private telephone service in his neighborhood, so she knew he would have to go to the corner and stand in line. She waited patiently. When he came back, he said, "I have something to tell you. I'm not really in love with you."

She focused right away on the phone call. Whom did he call? Did the conversation change his mind, or was it irrelevant? "I felt like if I could only figure out what was wrong about that phone call, that would have made it all right again," she said.

She went back to Stuttgart in disbelief. She could barely get herself out of bed each morning to drag herself to her office. "It was paralyzing," she said.

All she could think was that she needed to talk to him. She sent letter after letter asking him to call her. The mail service was fast and reliable throughout Germany, so she knew he was getting all her letters. She imagined that same phone booth, and all the people in line who would hear him as he spoke to her, witnessing what was going on between them. Perhaps these German strangers would recognize the injustice of it all, of this bright-eyed man who had romanced her and then, very suddenly, backed away. He didn't answer her letters and he didn't call. Two weeks later, his silence became so oppressive that Angela impulsively rushed to the train station and boarded the train to Berlin, an eight-hour trip.

She showed up at Heinrich's door at midnight. She was terrified that he wouldn't be home or that he would be with someone else. He answered the door alone. He set up a pallet on the floor and asked her to go to sleep. "I made a point of sobbing so long and so loud that he eventually came in to comfort me by having sex with me," she said. "Then he sent me away the next morning."

From an evolutionary perspective, Angela's dramatic journey was a demonstration of commitment, of the time and attention she was willing to devote to him: *See how much you mean to me? See what I can give you?* Rejection goads us to action despite the possibility of failure and stigma, because "being cut out of mating is an evolutionary dead end," Geher said. "That's why we see a lot of things in the mating domain that make people uncomfortable, that people see as difficult or strange. At the end of the day, mating is Darwin's bottom line."

Intense pursuit and expressions of need can force the beloved to heed his pursuer, shifting his attention and energy away from competing interests, sexual and otherwise. The pursuer's demanding presence may cause the target's other mating prospects to decide they'd rather not go through the trouble of dealing with an insistent rival. For these reasons, pursuit can sometimes succeed in winning back an estranged partner; adaptations have to work only some of the time to have staying power in a species. Angela's chase worked only as what evolutionary psychologists call a "short-term mating strategy": consolation sex with Heinrich.

Adding salt to the wound of rejection is the fact that the beloved's ability to turn you down in itself makes him more appealing. It's a sign of "high mate value." As Geher explained, "It's an ironic and not pleasant fact of human social life that not everyone's in a position to engage in social rejection, but when they do, it's immediately attractive. That person sees himself as having options."

The stakes in winning the rejecter rise. People who have been refused may "want that person even more because they perceive that person as having a higher mate value," he said. "But they are also thinking, 'Wow, this is going to help my confidence and assessment as a person and my own mate value if I can get the person to say yes.'"

Inasmuch as the impulse to nurture prospective offspring could make a woman a discriminating "chooser," once she's chosen, she may very well chase. J. D. Duntley, a professor of criminal justice and psychology at the Richard Stockton College of New Jersey, and David Buss, an evolutionary psychologist at the University of Texas at Austin, have published research theorizing that women engage in stalking primarily to prevent a partner from leaving or to get him back if he does leave. Men, they hypothesize, stalk for those reasons as well, but they are more likely than women to engage in "pre-relationship" stalking as a strategy to win a mate in the first place. Buss's extensive surveys on jealousy revealed that women reacted more strongly to emotional infidelity, in keeping with the evolutionary psychology theory that a partner's involvement with another woman siphons off his resources and attention. Men reacted more strongly to sexual infidelity, which could trick them into providing resources for offspring who aren't their own.

OUR REPRODUCTIVE SUCCESS may be the furthest thing from our mind. We use birth control (including methods such as implants and IUDs, which require attention only every few years), until we're ready for children—and then, increasingly, we rely on technologies from hormone shots to IVF to help us conceive. We may choose never to have children. Same-sex romantic pursuit, no less intense than hetero chasing, doesn't have the same direct link to reproduction. The lived connection between sex and childbearing is far looser for us than it was for our ancestors, even if the same genetic impulses course through us. Even Angela, who had unprotected sex and thus real reason to worry about potential offspring, wasn't consciously thinking about losing a possible father to her child. She mourned for the loss of his companionship to *her*. Without Heinrich, she remembered, the unmoored feeling in her life returned. "I had to get him back," she said. "It was an existential fear. I thought he was my lifeline. He really wasn't, but it sure did seem like it during that time."

We most often hear the psychological term "attachment" to describe the importance of a secure bond between parent and child for the child's survival and emotional development. But attachment has powerful benefits for adults as well. Romantic love holds out the promise of connection to a person who, in an echo of the parenting role, can provide an interchange of caregiving and attachment. It's what psychologists call a "secure base for exploration," promoting feelings of safety and confidence that allow partners to engage in the world in a focused and secure way.

Neuroscientists, in fact, are finding that both parent-infant bonds and adult couples work from the same motivational systems in the brain. Men and women react to separation and loss much as children (and, for that matter, other baby mammals) do. Their bodies gear up for pursuit. Heart rate and body temperature go up. The abandoned mammal is vigilant, stressed, and unable to sleep, its entire body geared toward reestablishing attachment. It's what psychiatrists Thomas Lewis, Fari Amini, and Richard Lannon identified as the "protest response," activated when emotional attachments are ruptured. We can focus on little else. "The drive to reestablish contact is sufficiently formidable that people often cannot resist it, even when they understand that the other person doesn't want anything to do with them," the authors write in *A General Theory of Love.*

This basic response doesn't vary significantly by gender. Brain scans of men and women who have been rejected recently look similar, said psychology professor Arthur Aron, who was part of the team of researchers on Helen Fisher's landmark brain-scan studies on people in love and after romantic rejection.

What may make a difference in whether the lovelorn follow through on the urge to chase are childhood trauma and attachment style. Neglect, physical abuse, and sexual abuse early in life increase the likelihood of criminal stalking and soft stalking—unwanted pursuit behaviors (UPBs) that characterize obsessive relational intrusion, but are less extreme than criminal stalking. People who have what's called an anxious (also known as preoccupied, ambivalent, or insecure) attachment style are more given to experiencing unrequited love. And as several studies show, they're more inclined to engage in UPBs after romantic rejection in both opposite-sex and same-sex scenarios.

One study revealed a majority (58 percent) of pursuers were classified as insecurely attached. The markers of insecure attachment are obsessiveness, insecurity, and moodiness in relationships. People with an insecure attachment style have high expectations of love. When they're in a relationship, the partner's attention is never quite enough. They have trouble making relationships last, or they're given to serial unrequited attractions, always seeking someone they can't have. "More anxiously attached people place a lot of importance on relationships and place their identity on these relationships," said Leila B. Dutton, one of the study's authors and a professor of criminal justice at the University of New Haven. "Relationships are more significant to them than to someone with a secure attachment style."

Her study found that another, equally significant predictor of pursuit is how much distress the rejected lover feels over the loss of the relationship. The level of hurt, anger, frustration, resentment, loneliness, and jealousy all contribute to the likelihood of pursuit. Someone who has a generally positive view of herself and others and is usually comfortable with intimate relationships could end up a needy chaser if her emotional investment in the relationship is sufficiently fraught. A recent major personal loss, such as a death or a prior breakup, may be a contributing factor. And if rejection occurs in a situation that's antagonistic to the relationship in the first place—such as a same-sex couple marginalized in a predominantly straight community—unwanted pursuit is more likely to happen. "Someone who is otherwise a fine and healthy person may try to get someone back and participate in unwanted pursuit because of the circumstances, even though they would say the behavior is uncharacteristic for them," Dutton said.

WHILE THE PROTEST response can push the unwanted woman to behave in ways she may regret, it's important to acknowledge the life-preserving impulses the reaction embodies. You're not only protesting rejection, you're also protesting the emotional and physical body blow it can entail. The next emotional stage after the protest response is despair, a physiological state that can include lethargy, loss of appetite, and profound sadness. Rejected lovers react very much like people suffering physical pain, or grieving over the death of a loved one. Forty percent of rejected lovers show signs of depression. Women are more inclined toward anxiety and depression than men, while men are more likely to resort to substance abuse. The finality of a breakup is rougher on young unmarried women, whose mental health tends to decline more than their male counterparts (who, interestingly, have a harder time than women when *ongoing* relationships get stressful); researchers speculate that, despite all the changes in women's social and economic status, a woman's identity and self-worth may still be overly tied up in having a man.

Overall, the loss of love can affect sleep and weaken our immune response. Though the end of a relationship shouldn't be fatal, it can be; it is a leading factor in suicide. We're more vulnerable to social isolation, which increases death rates among heart and cancer patients and heightens the risk of illness or death. That's not to say that winning over an estranged beloved, or even having a committed partner, is the only way to a healthy existence. But the protest response is linked to our survival instincts and our need to have a caring social support system.

Though the unwanted woman's chase might be in vain, it offers her a way to ward off this cascade of misery. "Getting on the train to go see him, that was my first happy moment," Angela said. "I thought I could get him back. I could get my life back. I felt powerless, and I took action."

I have listened to many stories like Angela's, of women who took action to protest rejection. I'm struck by the rebellious freedom of getting on that train. There's an emotional honesty in these moments—the unwanted woman is *doing something* instead of sinking into despair. She is swept up by instinct, by the profound human need for attachment, which the era of romantic practicality has tried to reduce to a game.

I know I should be moved only so far. The journey of the chase, whether it is a daylong train ride across Germany or years of effort to win a beloved, may take us away from our hopelessness. But once we confront a beloved and his refusal to love, we face a new set of questions. How vigorously do we protest?

Maggie, a thirty-six-year-old country singer and songwriter, was raised with the message that she could pursue what she wanted in life with just as much determination as a man. Her grandfather was a sanitation worker in Brooklyn, and her father started working at age nine delivering newspapers. He shined shoes, joined the army, and struggled his way into the middle class, becoming an accountant. As he brought up his own children in relative comfort, he tolerated few excuses from either Maggie or her older brother. "I was raised never to give up," she said. "You were supposed to just keep trying."

When her boyfriend of three years left her abruptly, she felt she had to do something to get him back. She came up with the most romantic gesture she could think of: She would serenade him with love songs. She rehearsed a set list of Johnny Cash tunes with a fiddle player and another singer to harmonize. Her gesture was a traditionally male one, but she didn't think about it that way. "I believed in the power of music. I wanted to come back with that redeeming quality," she said. "I thought, 'If I don't try, I'll never know if I could have gotten back with him, and the worst thing that could happen is that I'll feel as awful as I'm feeling now.'"

Her ex left town for three weeks, during which her plans for the ensemble fell through. She prepared to serenade him alone. He had always loved her music. She fantasized that the moment he heard her, he would remember that he loved her.

She knew he worked an overnight shift once a week, changing the displays at a gourmet supermarket. He was living with his parents, so serenading him after work was the only way to find him alone. The first week he was back, she drove by the store during his usual shift and saw his car there. She waited in the parking lot until he emerged at sunrise. The moment she walked toward him with her mandolin, she realized her plan wasn't going to work. She began to play anyway. He stopped her. "I can't hear that right now," he said. "It's over." He got in his car and drove off.

Not giving up staved off her hopelessness and despair for a while. But her persistence also obscured what I call The Line. The Line is the often blurry boundary between trying hard and trying *too* hard. It's the divide between courtship and aggression, between striving and violating someone else's life. However well intentioned Maggie's idea was, she was so absorbed in her plot that she couldn't see that confronting her ex alone in a parking lot before dawn might come across as disturbing rather than romantic. Romantic pursuit may be just as natural a tendency for a woman as for a man, but both have to face the same question: How ardently can you protest rejection without crossing The Line?

WHEN SYLVIA, THIRTY-FOUR, an editor, met Joseph, she had recently broken off her engagement to another man. The split wasn't traumatic. She had gradually realized that they didn't have as much in common as she once thought. She knew she didn't want to live permanently in France, where he was from. She moved to Chicago, ready to set up her own adult life in the city she loved. She planned to find a steady job, establish deep roots, and find someone she felt more compatible with.

From the first time Sylvia spotted him at a cocktail party, Joseph impressed her as exceptionally charismatic. "All the eyes in the room gravitate toward him," she said. "He wants everyone's attention and thrives on it." Yet when they were one-on-one, he listened intently. They had a similar sense of humor, both silly and cutting. What was missing with her French fiancé, that sense of common interests, was there right away with Joseph.

In the two years Sylvia and Joseph were together, though, he was never fully hers. At times she was certain he was gay. The first several times they tried to have sex, he couldn't keep an erection. He told her that once, in college, he'd taken Ecstasy and fooled around with a man. He dwelled on her physical descriptions of her past male lovers. She watched him let men hit on him, and he would flirt back. Sylvia was also tormented by his furtive pull toward other women. She discovered he'd lied about where he was on a Saturday night so he could go out with a girl he once slept with. He took several trips overseas to visit other women and never invited her. She was sure he had affairs. By the end of their relationship, she said, he never seemed to tell the truth. "He would lie about what was in a drawer in his apartment," she said.

When they split up, their mutual friends flocked around Joseph, who avoided her and portrayed her as the bitter one. "All my friends dumped me except this one girl," she said.

She went to dinner with the remaining friend. Sylvia drank too much wine and found she couldn't stop herself from venting her anger. "I was trying to explain why this guy was so awful and why I'd felt so betrayed," she said. "The more incidents I described to her, the more the bad stuff kept piling up."

In the wake of the breakup, she had been calling Joseph a lot, trying to learn the reasons he lied and kept her at an emotional distance. Their conversations often escalated into arguments. He never gave her satisfying answers. At dinner with her friend, she called again to berate him. He hung up on her. She kept calling back. "I knew I was going to a bad place," she said. "I told my friend, 'This isn't good. I've got to go home, chill out, watch a movie, and get back to myself.'"

At home, nothing helped. No matter what movie she watched, she saw manipulation. Even *Young Guns II*, a 1980s Brat Pack Western that always cheered her up, couldn't distract her. "I tried to read a book. No matter what I did, I couldn't stop feeling blindingly angry. I thought, I wasn't going to get rid of my anger until I dumped it on the person who deserved it."

Around two a.m., she took a cab to Joseph's apartment and knocked on his door to wake him up. She demanded he listen to her. She collapsed into a chair, half sitting on a note pad he'd left there. She looked at what he'd written. "There was this big long emotional letter to this girl he'd known earlier in his life," she said. "He hadn't been in touch with her for five years, but then he was writing about how he wanted to visit her in California. It was only three weeks after we'd broken up. It put me over the edge. He had no pity, no regret, no shame for all of this horrible stuff that he had done to me."

She yelled at him to tell her the truth about himself. She slapped him in the face. "Don't do that," he said. He threatened to call the police. "Go ahead," she retorted.

When the police arrived, she was crying so hard that she couldn't answer their questions. Joseph told them he didn't want them to arrest her. He just wanted her to leave. An officer guided her by the shoulders into the squad car to take her home.

The radio was set to a lite FM station playing a love song. "How could you play a song like that?" she protested. "Can't you see how terrible this is?" The police officer told her he wanted to cover up the sound of her weeping and she should calm down.

"You don't understand," she protested. "He cheated on me, and *I'm* the one who gets arrested!"

"At least you got a pop in before you had to leave," he chided her.

That night wasn't the last time Sylvia felt intense anger at Joseph. But it was the last time she confronted him about it. "I would think back to that night and say, 'That's not you. Try to let the past be past.'" Her determination to get some kind of justice for herself didn't get her anywhere. She was never going to learn the truth about Joseph's life. He was never going to acknowledge the pain he'd caused her.

When Sylvia thinks back to the confrontation with Joseph, she is struck by the rage she felt at her powerlessness. His withdrawal sent her back to some all too familiar childhood feelings. "I grew up with difficult parents, and I often felt my emotional needs weren't met by them," she said. When Joseph first came into her life, he gave her more support than she'd ever known. "He put on this show of 'I want to make you the happiest woman in the world,'" she said. "It was the first time someone worked so hard to make me think he would meet my needs, and then he turned into a shape-shifter. He shut off like a steel trap."

She remembers vividly a moment, in the heat of their argument, when she saw herself reflected back through his eyes. "I was that crazy psycho bitch that every man imagines lives inside of every woman," she said.

THE "CRAZY PSYCHO BITCH" haunts many of us as we contend with rejection. The primal frustration we feel gives us little real power to get love back, or to get a satisfying explanation of what went wrong. Yet the Psycho Bitch continues to protest, refusing to let her beloved get away with ambivalence, bad behavior, and the emotional blow of abandonment. She has the determination of a heroine, but she goes too far. Her disturbing persistence is a distortion of the Protestant work ethic/equal opportunity ideal: If you try hard enough, you can get what you really want. The Psycho Bitch embodies both the fierceness and the shame of being a woman who can't accept rejection and move on.

There are reasons why the Psycho Bitch surges forth. Sylvia had lost the man she thought would provide the love and care she always yearned for and didn't get as a child. Her protest response was sharpened by frustration at how withholding Joseph could be, along with the evolutionary challenge of jealousy; his attention and resources went elsewhere. Neurobiologically, when people realize that a reward—love, sex, drugs—isn't going to happen, the brain's network for rage, which is closely connected to areas in the prefrontal cortex that assess and expect rewards, is triggered. Unfulfilled expectations can make us furious and aggressive; animals denied an expected pleasure will bite or attack.

Mark Ettensohn, a Sacramento-based psychologist, says that overwhelming stress and anger can cause otherwise stable people to temporarily lose control. "Ideally, we develop a broad range of ways of dealing with adversity, and we can move fluidly between them and choose the right tool for the right situation," he said. "When life throws us a series of curveballs, those defenses can be overwhelmed. You can fall back into a more primal way of dealing with the world."

Sylvia's story brings up what's troubling about explaining romantic pursuit. Chasing may be an unconscious urge inherent to the perpetuation of the species, but we also have to acknowledge what happens when pursuit goes awry and becomes intrusive. The urge to protest rejection and run after love may be just as innate to women as it is to men. But that means that women have to contend with the implications of chasing too hard. Sylvia was standing, as I had stood, right on The Line, where objection blurs confusingly with violation.

5

Falling from the Stars

LOSING YOURSELF TO THE

NARCISSISM OF UNREQUITED LOVE

❦

THE LOWEST POINT OF MY OBSESSION
began when B. put aside the baseball bat and
let me into his apartment. I told him I was too
distraught to leave his side. He relented. We
took a long walk on the wooded trail of Frick
Park. It was right before Thanksgiving and the
park was nearly deserted. From time to time I
would stop him and put my arms around him,
trying to break through his reserve, but it was
like embracing a statue. He wouldn't hold me,
and he wouldn't look into my eyes.

In the late afternoon, we ended up in my
apartment. He let me touch him, and he touched
me back. At first what we were doing felt opti-

mistic, as if it could bring us to something healthy and right, freeing him from his confusion and me from my obsession. But then a sense of despair came between us. Was he with me only because I had begged him to be? He didn't want to enter me. Half-undressed, we gave each other orgasms. The intimacy was not a victory. It was an empty room, a mountaintop with no view, a holy grail made out of tinfoil. It was barren and sad.

He told me he had to return to his apartment and pack. He was catching a train the next morning to Washington, D.C., where he would spend Thanksgiving with his girlfriend and her family. Stunned, I watched him go.

The next morning, I went downtown alone to rent a white Kia. Several times during the eight-hour drive to my family Thanksgiving in Connecticut, I pulled off the highway to call B. from pay phones. I left long messages explaining why we should be together. I begged him to call me, to see me, to let the relationship that was supposed to happen between us finally begin. End it with her, I urged his voicemail.

I could barely speak to my family over the holiday. I buried myself in the work I'd gotten behind on, sneaking away from time to time to leave more messages. I couldn't stop myself. I didn't know what direction my life would go if he were not in it. I kept calling even though the words I spoke began to sound ugly, not because I threatened him—I never did—but because I was so needy. My future seemed incomprehensible. My pride was gone. Every message embarrassed me. I wanted to take back the words as they emerged. I think I said as much, awkwardly, on one of the messages. If he loved me back, I knew, I would be different, my power and my allure restored. But that wasn't happening.

I seemed to have sacrificed my entire being to an impossible love.

❦

MANY OF THE women I've surveyed and interviewed about unrequited love testify to this dark shift when they became someone
they couldn't recognize. They neglected their work. They isolated
themselves. They ate too much or too little. They smoked, drank,
took drugs, cut themselves, and engaged in other risk-taking behaviors. More than half of the women in my online survey said they
felt like they were losing their mind. "It ate up years of my life and
energy," wrote a thirty-five-year-old public health administrator
from New Mexico. "My life had become sad and small due to my
obsession." A forty-three-year-old student recounted, "I couldn't
eat, I couldn't sleep, I almost failed my courses. I broke my husband's heart." Talia Witkowski, a Los Angeles–based psychologist,
described herself in her teens and twenties as a kind of serial unrequited lover. She once traveled to Shanghai to be with a man she'd
had a fling with, even though he warned her that he was seeing
someone else and didn't want her to visit. She spent the trip in a
depressed funk and drank heavily. Her obsessions felt "like slavery,
like I'd been overcome by a kind of monster," she said. "Nothing
mattered but having the person return my love. I became extremely manipulative, compromised my integrity and morals, just
to get him to have sex with me. There was no pleasure in it."

Unrequited love, as we've seen, often revolves around what we
imagine the beloved to be and how loving him makes us see the
world in new ways. The revelatory potential of unrequited love lies
in our ability to step back and recognize what is motivating our
yearning. When the unwanted woman loses herself to unrequited
love, she can't separate herself from her fantasies about the beloved
and their future together. In this state, the love means everything
to her, and seems to merit every effort, no matter how hurtful or
self-destructive. This can seem like martyrdom. She feels she's doing it all for him. But this state of abjection is a profoundly narcis-

sistic one. It's all about her and her investment in the fantasy of love that she has created.

NOTHING ILLUSTRATES THIS state more vividly than the saga of astronaut Lisa Nowak. Nowak had a three-year extramarital affair with William Oefelein, an astronaut colleague. The romance ended when he informed her in a crowded NASA gym that he'd fallen in love with another woman. Three weeks later, Nowak drove nine hundred miles from Houston to Orlando, wearing an adult diaper so she wouldn't have to stop to urinate. Then she donned a dark wig and a trench coat and followed Oefelein's new girlfriend, Air Force Captain Colleen Shipman, through a parking garage. When Shipman refused to talk to her, Nowak attacked her with pepper spray.

And so Nowak became the "astro-nut," driven crazy by "lust in space," inspiring one-liners such as this one by Jay Leno: "She went to court yesterday and was released on her own incontinence." The media merrymaking reflected an all too common reaction to female stalking. Laughing is a way to shake off how frightening it is, a way to feel in control when faced with the prospect of a woman gone haywire.

Nowak's stalking *was* scary, and it could have been worse—just before she was arrested, she was seen stuffing in the trash a bag containing a loaded BB gun. She was carrying a four-inch buck knife and a steel mallet. The attack traumatized Shipman, who pleaded for a restraining order and testified in court about living in a constant state of fear. (Shipman and Oefelein are now married and running a freelance writing and photography business in Alaska.) The incident also put NASA under intense scrutiny. How could a woman so emotionally unstable not only have been sent into space the year before—but also be slated to be the voice of Mission Control for the next scheduled shuttle flight?

The fact is that before the breakup with Oefelein, Nowak showed little indication of being out of control. She had spent most of her career proving herself worthy of being chosen for a space mission, juggling long days and rigorous training regimens with raising three children. Earlier in her career, she applied six times to get in to the navy's test pilot school. One reason she kept being denied was that her legs didn't meet the minimum length requirement. She challenged the policy, which disproportionately affected women, and finally got in. After she was chosen to become an astronaut, she had to respond to reporters who queried her about daring to aspire to space travel when she had kids at home. "Anything you do is risky," she calmly told them. In 2003, not long after she found out she was scheduled for an upcoming space mission, the *Columbia* exploded, killing her best friend, Laurel Clark, and the rest of the crew. Nowak buried her own sense of loss—and her rising fears about meeting the same fate—by throwing her energy into helping Clark's family through their grief. The mission she was scheduled for was canceled as NASA tried to figure out what went wrong. During this acutely stressful time, Nowak's affair with Oefelein began.

When Nowak did go on the 2006 *Discovery* mission, her role required the utmost in focus. She was one of two "robo-chicks" assigned to operate the controls of the robotic arm that would allow the crew to examine the underside of the spacecraft for damage. One moment of inattention and the arm could swing wildly in the weightlessness of space, endangering the shuttle and its crew. She did her job well, and the *Discovery*'s successful mission provided the world with more proof that NASA had bounced back from the *Columbia* disaster. After the *Discovery* landed, Nowak toured elementary schools; made a triumphant appearance at her alma mater, the U.S. Naval Academy; and sat for an interview with *Ladies'*

Home Journal. She was slated to be on the cover of the May 2007 issue celebrating motherhood.

After Nowak's February arrest, several of her NASA colleagues felt, along with the shock of what she'd done, the loss of a valued colleague. Laurel Clark's widower, Dr. Jon Clark, a former NASA flight surgeon, became one of several NASA colleagues who expressed support for Nowak. He described her as having been "wonderful" and "nurturing" in his family's time of grief. In a letter to the Florida judge deciding Nowak's case, Clark said that astronauts could be vulnerable to depression from a "let-down period after the tremendous high of flying in space." Nowak's downfall was a collective loss. The *Ladies' Home Journal* cover was canned before the issue went to press. That über working mom at the pinnacle of human achievement was gone. And she had been *ours*—a product of our space program, our tax dollars, our progress on getting women into the most demanding and competitive professions, and our ongoing impractical desire to watch our fellow human beings go beyond the earth's gravitational pull.

The scandalous titillation of Nowak's ruin obscured the importance of these losses and how very sad her downfall was. The morning of her arrest, Nowak sat in the Orlando police department, utterly bewildered. She repeatedly insisted that what she had done wasn't normal for her. She was a good woman, a woman of accomplishment. "How could this be happening to me?" she asked. As exceptional as Nowak's life was, her bafflement is something any woman who has ever lost herself to unrequited love can relate to.

When Nowak was six, she watched Neil Armstrong step on the moon and knew she wanted to become an astronaut. So many children have this dream. They look at the glittering dome of the night sky and want to *be there*. She was one of the rare ones who made it. And then she fell, hard and fast, from the stars.

***

WHY DOES OBSESSIVE love have this power? Its neurochemistry gives us some basic insight: The addictive, reward-seeking mechanism of passionate love becomes more extreme. The unrequited lover is like a junkie, willing to do anything for a fix. She is flooded with feeling: fear, anger, guilt, shame, jealousy, and sadness. She has a goal she can't achieve. It hurts her, frustrates her, pisses her off. Nowak also saw a clear obstacle to her love: another woman. Dr. Louann Brizendine, the director of the Women's Mood and Hormone Clinic at the University of California, San Francisco, has commented that while it's normal to have rageful, jealous fantasies of hurting your rival, Nowak took the additional step of acting on them. Brizendine saw in Nowak's behavior signs that she was in a "fixed delusional state"—in which a clearly false belief (in this case, something along the lines of "If I attack my rival, I will get my lover back") seems indisputably true. Nowak was functioning normally in every other area of her life, yet lost her grip on reality—and self-control—when it came to coping with Oefelein's rejection. Other psychologists have speculated that Nowak had a personality disorder, which means that even though she functioned normally in everyday life, jealousy may have exposed disturbed patterns of thinking, feeling, and behavior underneath her hyper-achiever surface.

I would do anything for you. In mutual love, this line shimmers. With its connotation of self-sacrifice, the phrase seems a romantically extreme expression of commitment. But in unrequited love, the object—the "you"—doesn't want the commitment. So the expression becomes suspect, raising the question: What exactly is it that you're sacrificing yourself for?

The answer may lie in the complex dynamics of narcissism. The martyred unrequited lover sacrifices herself *to herself*—the self she believes will emerge from her beloved's attention, the noble creature trapped inside the suffering beast. The normal sort of narcissism that can emerge in passionate new love becomes entrenched and "highly emotionally charged," said forensic psychologist J. Reid Meloy. "You feel like you have a right to pursue this person, and you see yourself as different from other people. The greater your self-absorption, the less empathy you feel for others." This can be the beginning of a dangerous path, as Nowak's story shows: a "pathology of narcissism," in which the obsessed lover becomes acutely sensitive to rejection and feels shamed and humiliated by it, triggering the urge to retaliate.

AMBER, A THIRTY-EIGHT-YEAR-OLD aspiring actress in New Jersey, was in the Hudson County Correctional Facility on a drug conviction when she met Roy. The other women in her cell would get up on the sink and talk to men through an air vent. They urged Amber to try it herself. The man on the other side had a deep, raspy voice and spoke slowly. "I loved his voice," she said. "It sent chills through my spine."

They talked through the night. They discovered they were from the same neighborhood in Jersey City and knew a lot of the same people. Three days later, she saw a guy outside in the courtyard, doing triangle push-ups. He had dark skin, short hair, and a slim, muscular body. She found out it was Roy.

After she got out of jail, she visited him regularly and sent him money, "doing everything a woman was supposed to do." The day he was released, nearly a year after their first conversation through the vent, she waited eagerly for him to arrive. She sat on her porch late into the night, but he didn't show up. He rang the doorbell at eight the next morning. They slept together, an experience she described as "having sex, not making love"—as if all the affection he'd expressed while he was behind bars had never existed. He left soon after to go back to his ex-girlfriend, the mother of his daughter. "He was blowing me off," she said. "I couldn't believe how he made me feel after all the time I'd put into this." She had been sober for over a year but went out drinking that night.

In the ten years since, Roy has bounced in and out of jail, on and off heroin, and in and out of the relationship with his daughter's mother. None of this has stopped Amber from loving him. Her obsession with him has turned her life into an emotional version of the *Groundhog Day* movie. Every day she hopes he will change and be fully hers. When Roy is incarcerated, Amber is his only regular visitor. She writes him long letters every night, sends him money, and pays for his cell phone. Behind bars, Roy is expressive and warm. He promises to treat her right. But when he is released, instead of running into her arms, he starts using drugs again and pushes her away. She hangs on. Eventually, he's back in prison and the cycle of hope and disappointment begins again.

Amber knows she's living for the fantasy of a loving life with Roy, but she can't let it go. Her experiences in the here and now are not truly real or important, because Roy isn't with her. Her life is on hold.

Three years ago, Amber started living with another man. But whenever Roy is sprung and wants to be with her, she'll kick the man out or insist that Roy sleep on their couch. She loves her live-in boyfriend, "but I'm not in love with him. I told him to leave a billion times. I know my heart's not there for him. I told him to get someone who's there a hundred percent. What I want at the end of the day is Roy, the one I'm in love with. We are supposed to be together."

UNREQUITED LOVE CAN keep the unwanted woman in a "frozen state," said Suzanne Lachmann, a New York–based clinical psychologist. "How can she evolve or grow when her validation comes from a beloved who gives her so little?" Her hunger for attention is often rooted in her past. An unavailable father, for example, can lead a woman to fall for an unavailable guy later. It's a phenomenon that psychoanalysis calls transference—the redirection of feelings from a prior relationship, usually in childhood, onto a new person. "The reason you are doing it is out of a desperate hope for that person to repair that rupture within you," Lachmann said. At the same time, women who have sunk deeply in an unrequited obsession "don't feel deserving of reciprocity. They are so used to fighting for love that they blow up the meaning of even the slightest acknowledgment. In their lives, they didn't learn to want more, and they haven't had more."

However unsatisfying this frozen state is, it may seem more appealing than the alternative: facing what life is like without the dream of the man who's supposed to be yours. "The person can feel better when focused on the fantasy rather than stepping back and seeing the reality of a blighted life that's sad, lonesome, and full of loss," J. Reid Meloy said. "The hard work of mourning is avoided through obsessive thinking."

When obsessions become painful and entrenched, and the unwanted woman can't control the pull to be with her rejecting beloved, she enters what psychotherapist Rhonda Findling calls "the masochistic zone." Love becomes suffering. "You will do anything to keep the connection," she said. "You will sell your soul out, your pride."

Life in the masochistic zone doesn't seem anything like narcissism. The popular understanding of the term is that it entails vanity and selfishness. Narcissistic personality disorder (NPD) is characterized by grandiosity, an overwhelming need for admiration, and a lack of empathy for others. Psychologist Mark Ettensohn says this diagnosis captures only "half of the picture of narcissism." There's also "the flip side, which can include vulnerability, shame, fear of dependency, and a proclivity for feeling used, discarded, unimportant, and misunderstood. These are just as essential to narcissism as other traits." What both kinds of narcissism have in common is the tendency to use other people to fulfill parts of the self. When people with narcissism "feel like something is missing inside, they will look for it in another person, someone they idealize," he said. "And in the narcissist's mind, that person is experienced as an extension of the self. When that person disappoints the narcissist or fails to meet his or her expectations, the narcissist may savagely devalue the person they formerly idealized."

In turn, the other person may feel used. "They are unwittingly involved in a process the narcissist is using to feel okay in the world," Ettensohn said. "The narcissist's behavior cries out, 'Complete me!'" The unrequited lover overlooks her impact as she martyrs herself to love. She is in such pain that she can't reckon with the consequences of what she's doing. When the unwanted woman cries "I can't help it," she abandons her free will and her judgment, fundamental aspects of her humanity.

WHEN TILLIE, A retail buyer in northern Virginia, Googled Martin, she was fifty-one and hadn't dated since her painful divorce thirteen years before. She was too hurt by the end of her marriage and too busy raising her three children as a single mother. The idea of Martin, her ex-boyfriend from twenty-five years ago, simply "insisted itself" one day, for what felt like no particular reason. She discovered his blog. He had recently posted an article about losing his longtime job at a radio station in Colorado. It was the same job he'd had when they were together. She found out from earlier postings that he'd had a minor stroke the year before.

She hadn't planned on rekindling anything. She was worried about him and emailed him through his blog to find out whether he was okay. He wasn't. He called later that day to tell her that he had just gotten biopsy results back. He had a malignant lung tumor.

What followed that phone call was, as Tillie described it, three and a half months of romantic emails and long-distance conversations. She visited him once. She slept at a friend's home and spent her days with Martin. They took long drives on the scenic roads near his home and talked endlessly. They remained chaste, but the visit felt emotionally intimate. She is an observant Christian, and they spent a lot of time discussing spirituality. As his health continued to falter, she urged him closer to God and convinced him to reconnect with an estranged sister. He sent her roses on her birthday. She held out hope that he would recover and want a serious relationship with her. "Everyone wanted it to work out," she said, "It would have been a fairy tale."

But then the fairy tale went off-script. Martin had been doing well on chemotherapy, but the treatments started to wear him down. His breathing sounded labored. He told her he had gotten too weak to cook an egg. He still called her every day, but he sounded less patient. He made surly remarks to her. "I was feeling rejected," Tillie said. She tentatively asked if he thought they should take a break from the phone calls. He said yes and hung up on her. "We never spoke again," she said.

After that conversation, Tillie entered the masochistic zone. She pleaded with Martin not to cut her off. She left several messages on his phone. "I felt like I couldn't breathe," she said. "My stomach hurt. I said, 'Please call me, I feel ill!'"

He responded by email. She was crazy, he wrote, and he couldn't deal with her anymore. "I was trying to respect him, but I couldn't handle the hope of a future with someone and then have it snatched away," she said. "I felt such a sense of worth with him. I felt sick when that was yanked away."

A crisis counselor to whom she reached out through a twenty-four-hour mental-health hotline reassured her that her grief was justified, given how suddenly Martin had pulled away. However understandable her emotions, it's important to look closely at her reaction and the nature of her love for Martin. The distance between them and the additional limits of his illness left a lot of room for her fantasy to grow. All she had was his voice on the phone and a regular stream of emails to feed her ideas about how perfect they would be together. At first they both benefited. He needed her support. She got a lot out of being supportive. The relationship gave her an outlet for her strengths: her insight and her compassion. As so many unrequited lovers do, she tied up the prospect of a more serious relationship with a critical life goal: ending her long years of loneliness and single-mother martyrdom. Initially, her love seemed to be headed to that starry future. Even if their romance were curtailed by his death, she would be his final love, a grace in his last days.

When Martin cut off contact with her, he disrupted that fantasy. "To come that close to the dream of my heart and have it taken away from me was overwhelming," Tillie said. As she was swept up in the protest response of the newly abandoned, she lost perspective. Her "sick feeling" took precedence over his worsening cancer, as if her life were ending, too. She described the end of their relationship in fatal terms: "To open up to someone again and have him kill you was hard." She was swept up in what Meloy calls the "sense of entitlement" that can emerge from fantasies about the beloved.

Tillie told me that after a few days, she gave up and stopped calling him. But she held out hope that he would get better and reconnect. He sent her two curt emails informing her of his worsening condition. A few months later, Martin's ex-wife told Tillie that he was dead. At his funeral, a friend of his told Tillie how important she was to him after he got his diagnosis, and this news gave her some peace. "I couldn't let him go until he died," she said. "After that, there was no possibility that he was going to call me."

IN THE LITERARY realm, self-sacrifice in its most extreme form—suicide—seems the ultimate expression of unrequited love. The publication in 1774 of Goethe's *The Sorrows of Young Werther*, the story of a man who kills himself over his obsession with a woman who marries someone else, caused a rash of copycat suicides. Some of the men who killed themselves were found dressed like Werther, or with the book open to the passage detailing his death. Germaine de Staël's 1802 epistolary novel, *Delphine*, overtly presents its protagonist as a female Werther, grappling with an *amour-passion* that is suffocated by the social priorities of the day. Delphine takes poison when she finds out the fiery Spaniard she loves is sentenced to death for his association with the old regime in revolutionary-era France. This kind of plot line comes from the Romantic era's lionization of extreme states of feeling and political heroism. Suicide is imagined as a mystical release from social oppression and romantic disappointment.

The fascination over suicides caused by unrequited love became a full-blown cliché in the Victorian era. Stories of pining suicidal women were common in broadsheets and annuals. They were figures of pity, victims of men who had more status, power, or strength than they did. In "The Suicide," a poem in a holiday annual, Ida, abandoned by her beloved in favor of a wealthier bride, walks into the sea to drown herself: "A plunge was heard—a dying groan /

—A bubble in the moonbeam shone." The trope of the suicidal un-wanted woman, which persisted despite the fact that women had a lower suicide rate than men, reinforced the idea of the emotionally dependent woman. If a man was to be a woman's main reason for living, losing him was portrayed as a reason to end her life. These stories also served as cautionary tales, since the economic and po-litical reality of the time was that many women couldn't live much of a life without a man. Unless they came from substantial privi-lege, they'd risk drowning in poverty and social stigma.

This risk is much diminished today. Yet even in the era of ro-mantic practicality, there's plenty of intrigue with the idea that sui-cide is the supreme gesture of lovelorn recklessness. I've listened to a car full of tween girls belting out Bruno Mars's "Grenade," a pop song about catching an explosive and diving in front of a train for the sake of a hard-hearted beloved. When I asked them about it, all of them agreed vehemently that this sort of behavior was "stu-pid." No one will develop self-destructive urges just because a tune on the radio makes it sound catchy. But the song and those sui-cide narratives of yore do tap into something real. If the unwanted woman gets mired in the delusion that her beloved's attention is the only thing that validates her, the lack of it could send her into a precariously fragile state.

CAROLYN, TWENTY-FOUR, CAME from a conservative Christian family in western Pennsylvania. As she entered adulthood, she fell away from the religion and started to come out as a lesbian. Two of her siblings refused to eat with her, quoting a Bible passage from Corinthians that admonishes the faithful not to take meals with unbelievers. Another sibling stopped talking to her. She lived in fear that her parents supported her only out of a sense of Christian duty to see her through college. Once she earned her degree, she worried, they would disown her.

At college, she found herself in a completely different world. She studied film and animation at an elite art school in New England. Most of her fellow students struck her as snobbish, unwilling to be friendly because she was slightly older. In class discussion, she perceived them as competitively pretentious. One afternoon during a break in her directing class, she exchanged exasperated glances with Gus, a classmate. "It was like, 'Oh, please, we have to go back in and face those people.'" He seemed a kindred spirit and her heart jumped.

They became friends and worked on films together. The last day of class, everyone presented a final project. She was startled to see that Gus's film was full of references to her life. He knew she loved 1980s music and YouTube videos of owls, and she often complained to him that she had a terrible memory. The film featured a female character in an owl mask, dancing to 1980s music. Later in the film, Gus's character, speaking off-screen, asks the dancer, "Do you remember we did this?" She replies, "I don't remember what you're talking about."

Carolyn didn't say a word during the discussion that followed. "But then I was like, 'He knows what he did,'" she said. "He made this person based off of me to show me how much he loves me. I convinced myself of that." She was euphoric.

She spent hours on social media, reading every tweet and status update he posted. She read all his "likes" and "favorites." She posted as much as she dared on his Facebook wall, messaged him ideas and links, and sent out tweets in hopes that he would respond. "I would obsess over what I was going to say to him to make sure it was perfect," she said. "I felt this terror that I was going to say something wrong. I wasn't messaging him constantly, but I spent a lot of time figuring out what I was going to say. I'd be lying in bed, taking a shower, getting coffee, and thinking about what I should post next."

She wanted him to see that she was different, so he would want to be with her. What exactly she desired was hard to define. She knew he was also gay. "It was another thing we had in common," she said. Sometimes she would fantasize about kissing him, though she didn't want to sleep with him. Her focus was on his eyes, his face, and his words, not his body. "I fantasized about us living together and having a close intimate relationship, but not a sexual relationship. I would be his one true friend. Other people could have sex with him, but we would always be together," she said. "I wanted him to be a part of my family, a family that I would make."

Carolyn spun a dire web of meaning around Gus. She wanted him to be family because her own family was rejecting her—but he couldn't offer her that closeness. When he didn't respond to the ideas she emailed and texted, she was devastated. She stopped looking for traffic before she crossed the street. She drove to the ocean and, just like the tragic heroine of "The Suicide," walked into the frigid water; a sandbar prevented her from going out too far. Another time, she got drunk and walked to an abandoned drawbridge on the outskirts of the city in the middle of the night. The bridge had been stuck in the open position since it went out of use in the 1970s. She climbed to the top of the open bridge and walked on the narrow ledge, high above the river. She told herself she was daring fate. If she fell, that meant she was supposed to die.

The myth that fictions such as *Werther* and "The Suicide" perpetuate is that romantic rejection alone leads to suicidal behavior. Though the loss of love is a common factor, a central principle of mental-health risk management is that untreated depression is the main cause, and no single life event can be pinpointed as the only trigger for suicide. Carolyn's self-destructive impulses were at the center of many risk factors: She was socially isolated and had a tenuous connection to her family. She was impulsive and sensitive and struggled with depression. She was drinking. And she took Gus's silences as a rejection of who she was.

Finally, Carolyn found a way to express what she was feeling instead of using it against herself. At the end of the school year, she offered to drive Gus to the airport. They met for breakfast beforehand, and she gave him a diary full of love poems. "I had to do something," she said. "My feelings were driving me crazy. It had been this secret. I thought that if he was aware of how I felt, then I could deal with it." She didn't see him at all over the summer. When they saw each other at school, he didn't say anything about the diary. Instead of being devastated, she realized at last that the relationship she dreamed of wasn't going to happen. She was no longer consumed with provoking responses from him, and the drawbridge no longer called to her.

Carolyn and I first spoke about a year after her obsession ended. I followed up with her three years later. She was living in Colorado, far from her western Pennsylvania hometown, but she told me that her relationship with her parents had improved. They hadn't disowned her, as she had feared. We talked about how her obsession with Gus had changed her approach to relationships. She said she now handles rejection in a much more stable way. She's learned to be wary when someone makes her feel the way she first felt with Gus—elated and suddenly confident. "I take a step back and think, 'Why do I feel like that?'" she said. "I try to talk to the person and learn more about them." The process she described seemed to be about breaking down that initial powerful narcissistic fantasy. The person she's attracted to, she now realized, won't complete her—and with her more reflective approach, she might be able to see that person more clearly.

FACING MY OWN narcissism has pushed me to consider something I couldn't consider when I was obsessed: the impact of my actions on B. It's likely he felt harassed and confused, beset by the moral dilemma of the rejecter. He very well might have felt violated, angry, frightened, or worse. I'll never know. After my obsession ended, I decided not to seek him out for any reason, though for a while our proximity meant we ran into each other occasionally. Even now, I suspect that wanting anything from him might come across as invasive—even (perhaps especially) the answer to the question of what my obsession felt like to him.

Yet I knew I needed a more comprehensive way to see outside the self-absorbed perspective of the unwanted woman who's lost herself to unrequited love. I've noticed in my survey responses, interviews, and casual conversations a strong tendency to see the beloved as the self-centered and sadistic tormentor who won't give you the relief of returning your love. Though cruel manipulators do exist, no matter the character of the rejecter, rejection will *feel* cruel and self-serving when you've got so much invested. I spent plenty of time when I was obsessed seething about what B. was "doing to me"—in retrospect, I don't think he was a cruel manipulator. He was confused and sometimes insensitive, but these are far lesser sins.

With this new understanding of the unrequited lover's self-absorption, I felt I had to look at the problem from the other side. When the unwanted woman loses herself to the narcissism of unrequited love, what is the impact on the beloved, who must witness her breakdown?

ᴡ

AFTER RENZO AND his girlfriend broke up, he spent a lot of time with a group of fellow South American expats living in Manhattan. The split was unexpected and painful, and he needed their support and company. One of the women, Yoselin, drew particularly close to him. "She took the role of good friend and mother, because she felt I was lost," he said.

She had a beautiful smile, and he told her so. They kissed and hugged every time they met. It was part of their culture, he said. He was affectionate with all his friends and generous with compliments to the opposite sex, and Yoselin was no exception. He walked her back to her apartment at the end of evenings out, in what he regarded as a gentlemanly gesture. When she fell ill with shingles, he stopped by her apartment every day to take care of her. He enjoyed her friendship, but he wasn't attracted to her.

Renzo, who is a composer, was so anguished over his breakup that he fell behind on writing a commissioned piece for a chamber orchestra. "I knew I had to reorganize myself," he said. He threw himself into finishing the work. One afternoon Yoselin stopped by his apartment while he was composing. He greeted her and explained that he had to keep working. She set about cooking a meal for him. After they ate, she asked him what else she could do to help him. He said she could mark measure numbers on the score. "I trusted her hand," he said. "She did it perfectly." He would come to regret accepting her offer of help. But at the time, he was absorbed in trying to finish the piece. "I just thought she was helping me, as I had helped her when she was sick," he said.

The evening the piece was performed, Yoselin "behaved as though she were part of the composer, as if she understood what I had gone through to write the piece, as if she knew what the piece was about," Renzo said. "It was as if she was my wife and part of the process. That did not go over well with me."

A few days later, he returned to his apartment to find his voice-mail full of messages from his friends, asking if he was okay. He noticed some of his papers were out of place. He discovered that Yoselin had convinced all their friends and the super of his apartment building that Renzo intended to kill himself in the bathtub. The super had let her into the apartment to check on Renzo while he was out. She came back later to tell him what she had done. "I got really mad, because it was an imposition and she was doing something that was not for her to do, out of some dream of the woman who helps the artist," he said.

Yoselin's calls and visits increased. She wrote letters to his siblings abroad. She even visited his parents, who lived near Renzo in Manhattan. Her message was twofold: She warned them that Renzo was emotionally and mentally weak. And she confessed to them that she could not live without him.

Renzo began to avoid his home. He had a first-floor apartment and knew she could see the light from the street whenever he was inside. He stopped going out with their group of friends. He was afraid to pick up the telephone. When he started dating another woman, Yoselin became even more distraught. She cried whenever she saw them together. One afternoon he was staring out his front window, as he often did, and saw her on the street. Their eyes met, and he felt he had to open the door. She handed him a bunch of flowers. Then she lay down on the floor and began to cry. Again and again she asked how he could be seeing someone else. "We had something that was so beautiful!" she protested. She sobbed and cursed and asked the same question repeatedly.

He sat on the couch and watched her. He tried to explain that they had never been more than friends, but he couldn't stop her lament or get her to leave. It was the first of several visits when she would lie prostrate in distress. Even though he knew he wasn't to

blame for her behavior, he regretted the encouragement he unwittingly had given: the affection, the compliments, and most of all,
his acceptance of her offer of help. "I should have used my eyes
better and been more careful," he said.

We can see through Yoselin's eyes the hope she placed in his
early affection and acts of kindness. Being cared for when you are
sick is a classic marker of intimacy and commitment—"in sickness
and in health," the wedding vows say. But that's also what good
friends do. Renzo saw his caretaking only as an expression of
friendship, which at the time he badly needed. Research on unrequited love shows that these different interpretations are very
common. One side values the growing friendship; the other reads
it as a buildup to romance. Yoselin's misreading grew to surreal
proportions—to the point where she deluded herself into believing
that Renzo wanted to kill himself and needed her to save him. This
is where she lost herself.

Even though Renzo hasn't seen Yoselin in fifteen years, the image of her on the floor keeps coming back to him. He remembers
the numbers on the clock as he went to let her in: 12:45. He remembers what she was wearing: a white shirt and a blue skirt. And
he remembers that she lay down right inside the door, as if she
couldn't go any farther. "I hated that," he said. Through his eyes,
we can imagine how excruciating it must have been to watch her
lying there. You would want to do anything to make her leave, but
in the face of so much vulnerability, there are no good options. "It
was difficult for me to see a person crumble like that, and become
something so small," he said.

Renzo could not be the person Yoselin fantasized about, the
lover-composer-compatriot-partner. In losing herself to the narcissism of unrequited love, she experienced this disappointment
so acutely that she couldn't, as Renzo so aptly put it, "see herself

again." But what happened to Yoselin was Renzo's loss, too. After his new relationship grew serious and eventually led to marriage, Yoselin left him alone. He was greatly relieved. Yet he also mourns for the Yoselin he knew before she lost herself. She was his friend and a part of the community that helped him out at a difficult time in his life. He had believed in the value of the warm ways of his homeland, embodied in her and the friends with whom they used to drink wine and go salsa dancing. "She had everything in her to be this wonderful human being," he said. Renzo could not be the person to restore her to her strengths. He hopes she found a way to do it herself.

6

The Gender Pass

FEMALE STALKERS AND THEIR
INVISIBLE VICTIMS

ᵥ

IN THE WAKE OF MY OBSESSION WITH B.,
I met a graphic designer and visual artist I'll
call Patricia. She was in her mid-fifties, with
expensively tinted blond hair. She had grown
up in Georgia and wore the air of a former
Southern belle, but with a proud, don't-mess-
with-me edge. One evening I told her about
my unrequited love and the lengths it drove
me to. "Honey," she said. "That was *nothing.*"

She proceeded to tell me about the affair
she began when she was thirty-nine. At the
time she was living outside San Francisco.
She was married and had a nine-year-old son.
Her family began to take sailing lessons, but

her husband didn't take to the sport. So she continued the lessons alone. She found sailing exhilarating. "I felt refreshed after a race," she said. "I'd spent myself physically, hauling sails, water in my face. It was much better than seeing a shrink, and cheaper, too."

One evening at the marina, she met a man she asked me to call Wolf, for his loner spirit and ruggedness. They had what she described as a strong intellectual rapport, which meant a lot to her. She had a college degree but had been raised to treat higher education as a means to find a husband. She had always felt insecure about her intelligence. Wolf, who lived in a converted tack house on a ranch, seemed to be everything her corporate husband was not.

The affair lasted over a year. He pressured her to leave her husband, but she refused. He grew insistent and aggressive. Once, he hit her so hard that she fell to the floor. Another time, he wouldn't let her leave his house until the next day. She had no way to explain her absence to her husband, who'd been terrified about her disappearance.

When Wolf told Patricia he didn't want to see her anymore, she couldn't accept it. She would go to the marina and lie in wait in his sailboat. She wrote fragments of Edna St. Vincent Millay poems in nail polish on the boat's beautiful wood: *I know what my heart is like / Since your love died.* She stole things from the boat, including a sail. "I became like a predator," she said. "I wanted to catch his scent, so I could feel near him."

When Wolf began to see someone else, Patricia was consumed with jealousy. At night, after her husband fell asleep, she snorted cocaine, got into her Jaguar, and sped the eighty miles to confront Wolf. The drive ended on dusty, windy roads. She would park out of earshot and tiptoe to the house. Before she walked in on him, she peed near his front door, "to make my mark."

She begged him to come back to her, but he resisted, telling her he was too involved with his new girlfriend. From time to time he would relent and spend a night or a weekend away with Patricia. She rented a studio on an estuary for the two of them to escape to, but he never showed up. She discovered that he had gone to Lake Tahoe with his girlfriend for her family reunion. The news sent her into what she described as attack mode. "You're going to find this person and confront him and nothing else matters," she said.

She found out where he was staying by calling resorts in Lake Tahoe and claiming to be part of the family reunion. She rented a car she knew Wolf wouldn't recognize. She gave her husband the bizarre excuse that she had promised his father she would go to Sacramento to research his family's genealogy. She said she didn't care if he went with her, so he did. When they passed Sacramento, she explained they would be staying in Lake Tahoe, even though it was over two hours outside the city. Her husband didn't stop her. By now he had found out about Wolf and had tried to get her to stop seeing him. Patricia knew she was hurting her husband, but she couldn't stop herself from her chase. "It was all about me," she said.

She rented a cabin near Wolf's. After her husband fell asleep, she went out to Wolf's cabin and began throwing rocks at it. She ran in circles, beating on the doors and the walls. "Come out! I know you're in there," she yelled. "You think you can do this to me? We had plans!"

A friend of Wolf's girlfriend came out and got into his car to go for the police. Patricia threw her body on the car hood to keep him from moving. She broke the windshield with a stick. He threw her off and drove away. She ran back to her cabin and told her husband they had to leave. After they got home, a police officer arrived with an arrest warrant. A restraining order was issued against her, and she had to pay damages for the smashed car.

In the weeks that followed, squad cars regularly cruised by her house—not to monitor her but to mock her. Police officers would roll down their windows, wiggle their tongues at her, and laugh. "The word was out," Patricia said. "I was a horndog, a loose woman, available. When it wasn't that at all."

She remained fixated on Wolf, her rage at his abandonment still vivid. She turned to her art to help her cope. She created a sculpture for an art show put on by the Guerrilla Girls, a feminist art movement pushing for greater representation of work by female artists. The piece, which she called *The Legend of the Lost Cause*, included a copy of Dante's *Inferno*, her police report, a photographic image of Wolf superimposed with a hyena face, and a railroad spike going through a flaccid cloth penis. She took her husband and son to the opening. "People were looking at me like 'This is your son, and he's looking at this?'" she remembered. "I was so self-absorbed. I failed to realize anyone else's feelings."

The sculpture and Patricia's pride in it underscore the obliviousness that can come over women who cross The Line and keep going, becoming stalkers. "The person appears to give little thought to their impact on the other," said forensic psychologist J. Reid Meloy. "That's how you can see the narcissism. They are dismissive or surprised when they're asked if they thought about the other person. In the most extreme cases, I hear things like: 'I don't care what he thinks! I'm going to have a relationship with him anyway.'"

Unrequited love can be a potent and revealing manifestation of the wish to escape from an unhappy marriage, oppressive social mores, and other constraints. But while Patricia hooked her anger to a feminist movement, there is nothing liberating or feminist about real-life stalking. Even though Wolf had wronged and abused her, Patricia's pursuit of him was itself invasive and violent. But like the cops who teased her after her arrest, we tend to resist seeing the actions of Patricia and other women who stalk as cause for alarm. We'd rather give female stalkers the gender pass, telling ourselves what they're doing is funny or nutty and not really a problem. It's far more comfortable—and comforting—to mock their actions than to reckon fully with their impact.

THE DARK SIDE of the urge to pursue, no matter which gender is doing the chasing, is its potential for harm. Romantic pursuit, as we've seen, falls along a continuum. At one end are courtship initiatives, with the risks, pleasures, and privileges of being the one who takes the lead. At the other is criminal stalking, which can ruin lives.

H. Colleen Sinclair, a psychology professor at Mississippi State University, has done extensive research on this continuum. For her, the movement from courtship to stalking is clear, no matter who is the perpetrator. At one end of the continuum are everyday efforts—flirting, attentive emails and texts, phone calls—to form a relationship or reconcile one. Then there are surveillance and monitoring behaviors, when pursuers' motivations are a blend of love and anger. All along the way, frequency and degree matter: Is it one text a day or a hundred? A dozen roses or a roomful of them? Then there are the most extreme measures: trespassing, threats, harassment, coercion, and violence. At this point, "there's no romance," she said. "They are doing this to hurt. Once they move from surveillance to aggression, the line isn't blurry."

Pursuers may tell themselves that their stalking is a form of love or courtship, she allowed, but that's "just like we used to talk about a rapist as the guy who is overwhelmed with passion." Today we have a similar myth about stalking. "People think it's about being so in love, you're not able to control yourself," Sinclair explained. "But you're driven by retaliation and obsession rather than love and idealization. Once you're aggressive, you're not idealizing. You're not in love. All that's left is the obsession."

Stalking is commonly seen as a crime against women, and for good reason. According to a 2010 National Intimate Partner and Sexual Violence (NIPSV) survey, women are three times more likely than men to have been stalked. That still means plenty of male stalking victims. One in nineteen men have been stalked, and about half reported their stalkers were female. The definition of criminal stalking varies somewhat from state to state, but the three main criteria for the crime are repeated, unwanted, and intrusive behaviors; implicit or explicit threats; and causing fear. The NIPSV study surveyed self-identified victims and was based on a definition of stalking that led them to feel "very fearful" or believe that they or someone in their life would be harmed or killed as a result.

But intent and fear are often not clear in the complex dynamics of unwanted romantic and sexual pursuit. Targets may not feel the level of alarm the NIPSV study assessed. They may not perceive themselves as victims, even when they feel harassed and afraid. Pursuers may not see themselves as wanting to cause harm. If we set aside these questions and again turn our focus to a softer definition of stalking, the gender disparity markedly diminishes.

Sinclair began to see this pattern emerge during her graduate studies in the 1990s, a time when anti-stalking laws were new. She'd gotten into the field out of an interest in what she had been calling "violence against women." She had done stints volunteering at a battered women's shelter and on a rape-crisis hotline. Yet the research she was working on, along with studies on other forms of relationship violence and abuse, was showing again and again that there were plenty of female aggressors and male victims, too many to see as aberrations. The idea that stalking was purely a matter of "patriarchal terrorism" didn't hold up. "It was a change in perspec-

tive," she said. "I don't refer to it as violence against women anymore. It's interpersonal violence or relationship aggression. Before,
it had always been seen as a women's issue."

Several peer-reviewed studies conducted since 2000 scrutinize
the question of gender and unwanted pursuit. The results show
that women are just as likely as men to engage in a number of
stalking tactics—and even *more* likely to resort to certain kinds.
In one study, approximately one third of women reported using
"mild aggression"—including threats, verbal abuse, and physical
abuse—after a breakup, compared to about a quarter of men. In
another set of findings on obsessive relational intrusion, the rate
of women who stole or damaged property was twice the rate of
men—and the rate of women who caused physical harm was almost three times higher. Female pursuers were just as likely
as male pursuers to resort to severe violence, such as kicking and
choking. Criminology researcher Carleen M. Thompson pin
pointed one possible reason that the level of female-perpetrated
relationship pursuit violence is so high: a sociocultural attitude
that is more disapproving of male violence against women than
female violence against men.

Women, the research suggests, are giving themselves the gender pass. They may be more likely to feel they have a right to their
behavior, while men, with the "chivalry norm" that stigmatizes
violence against women, are more likely to know that, at least in
principle, they shouldn't be getting out of hand. Researcher Leila
Dutton at the University of New Haven has considered the possibility that one reason the rates of female stalking behaviors are
so high is that women may feel less defensive about what they are
doing. That makes them more comfortable than men are about reporting their pursuit behaviors in a survey, even though their identity remains anonymous. "It's much less socially acceptable for a

man to hit a woman," she said. "We don't take women's violence as seriously, so women can get away with it."

This assumption is compounded by the widespread impression that female stalkers of male targets don't cause real harm. Research into perceptions of stalking scenarios finds that respondents view female stalkers as less dangerous and problematic than male stalkers. Male victims of female stalkers are seen as better able to defend themselves than female victims. It's not hard to guess why the perceived scariness of male stalkers might overshadow the impact of female stalkers. "Given that men have more privilege, power, size, and muscle, there's greater fear associated with their pursuit activities," said Jennifer Langhinrichsen-Rohling, a clinical psychology professor at the University of South Alabama who studies relationship violence. "But when we don't view female aggression as serious or noteworthy, women don't get feedback that their behavior is not okay." As several experts pointed out, the "privilege, power, size, muscle" rationale only goes so far once gender-neutral tools of the stalking trade enter the picture. How much weight a stalker can bench-press doesn't matter in cyberspace or once she has a pistol in her hand.

My own behavior with B. was never violent or threatening. But I was invasive. When he opened his front door in response to my compulsive knocking, the tight, guarded look on his face and the sharp tone in his voice surprised me. I had become something he felt he needed to defend himself against. It took me a long time to admit that my pursuit of B. could have been harmful. I saw what I was doing mainly as self-destructive. If I used the word "stalking" to describe my actions, it was always with some irony. It was only when I gender-flipped my experience that I could come to terms with what I did. When I envisioned a man acting as I had, I saw a creepy stalker, with nothing ironic about him.

In my discussions with researchers and clinical psychologists, I discovered that they found gender-flipping a persuasive tool in getting women and girls to face the implications of female stalking. In one of H. Colleen Sinclair's psychology classes, her students insisted that Tiger Woods's ex-wife, Elin Nordegren, was justified in allegedly chasing him out of the house with a golf club and causing his SUV to crash—until Sinclair asked them to consider how they'd feel if Tiger had been the one wielding a golf club in a jealous fury. In a relationship violence-prevention program run by Langhinrichsen-Rohling and colleagues for low-income pregnant teens in Mobile, Alabama, several girls told stories of aggressively tracking and confronting the fathers of their children. The girls defended their behavior on the grounds that they suspected the fathers were cheating on them or had new girlfriends. The others in the group agreed with this reasoning. They tended to see female vengeance as exciting. "They thought, 'Yeah, she was really taking it to him!'" Langhinrichsen-Rohling said. She countered by asking what they would think if they were listening to males telling the same stories. "Over and over I would pose hypotheticals and switch the gender, and we'd see perceptions change."

In my interviews with women whose pursuit crossed The Line between courtship and harassment, I found that their focus, like Patricia's, was usually on how they'd been wronged. They were seeking love, the truth, rightful retribution. They couldn't be hurting their beloved—he was the one hurting *them*. Psychotherapist Rhonda Findling, the author of *Don't Text That Man*, said, "They're so fixated on the other person, they don't even care about him. They don't care what he's saying." This narcissistic trance isn't unique to women. Yet while men fall into this trance despite strong social messages that warn them not be aggressive, women don't have these cautions. They may even use the stereotype of the male aggressor as a weapon in their pursuit.

LUKE, A FIFTY-FIVE-YEAR-OLD marketing director, first described Dara to me as "the porch diver." She had become a family joke, a story he hauled out regularly. "I look at the whole thing with mild amusement. It's funny. It's a party story."

He met Dara through an online dating service. They went out for margaritas. She told him that she had recently gone through a rough divorce. Her husband, she told Luke, had served her with papers when she was in the hospital, recovering from a serious accident.

At the end of the evening, Luke said in the noncommittal parlance of Internet dating that it had been nice to meet her. She replied with a question: "If you could ask me anything to do next, anything at all, what would you ask?"

"I'm a guy, and she's an attractive woman," he told me somewhat sheepishly. "So I said, 'Well, come home with me and go to bed with me.'"

She came home with him, went to bed with him, and didn't leave. She immediately assumed "all the trappings of a girlfriend," Luke said. She was possessive and insisted he get off the dating sites he frequented. She wanted him to stop talking to other women, even his friends. After two weeks, he told her she needed to go home.

She called him several times a day. He didn't pick up when he saw her caller ID, but sometimes she'd get to him through the office staff at work. "She'd be really hostile," he said. "Like, 'What are you doing, ducking my calls? You don't want to speak to me? Is that how little I meant to you?'" Luke's son played in a band, and Dara regularly showed up in the audience with her friends.

She came to his house early one morning to get some of her things. She pulled from his closet a few shirts she had bought him and grabbed some shirts that she hadn't.

"Some of those are mine," he said. "I'd like to keep them."

"They're all mine," she said. "You're not getting them."

He followed her out to his front porch, trying to get his shirts back. She started to scream. Then she threw herself down, face-first, on the tiled concrete porch floor. She stood up, her nose bleeding. "You hit me, you knocked me down!" she yelled. "I'm calling the cops." She dialed 911.

Two squad cars arrived. Luke and Dara gave their contradictory statements. He tried to stay calm, reasoning that the more rattled he acted, the more he'd seem like a domestic abuser. "I was pretty sure I was going to go to jail," he said. "I felt like you do when you're in traffic and someone smacks into your car."

The police were getting ready to take Luke in when a couple of his neighbors came out and told them they'd seen Dara hurl herself to the floor. The police offered Luke the opportunity to press charges against her for making a false report. Luke gave her the gender pass instead. "No," he said. "I just want her out of here."

He has since learned from Facebook (he didn't dare unfriend her) that she was seeing someone else, though she occasionally dropped hints in a status or a comment that she was still interested in him. Near the end of our conversation, he told me that he was in a new relationship, too. "I'm off the deep end with this one," he said. "I'm hoping she's the last love of my life." He confessed that he lived with a steady fear that what happened with Dara could happen again. "It's deeply affected me, even though I have a calm demeanor and try to take everything calmly."

What happened with Dara, then, was much more than a party story Luke could pull out for laughs. Dara and the hazard she represented was an ongoing source of worry, shaping his emotional landscape. The freewheeling divorcé's existence that he'd been living suddenly seemed treacherous.

The contrast between Luke's initial persona, of a laid-back guy who could brush off a one-night stand gone awry, and that of a man transformed by fear is emblematic of the contradictory state of the male stalking victim. A review of research on male victims of relationship-related stalking published in the *International Journal of Men's Health* in 2009 shows these men not only feel that they are less likely to be taken seriously, they also tend to take themselves less seriously. Men will describe stalking acts as frustrating or annoying rather than threatening or frightening. They are less likely to call themselves victims, and they are less likely to contact the police. Yet they confess to being changed by the experience. They may become more cautious and paranoid, or suffer from anxiety and shifts in their attitudes and personality. In these ways, male targets of female stalking are victims—but if no one wants to see them as such, they become invisible, even to themselves.

Langhinrichsen-Rohling has described several reasons why this is so. Men are generally less likely to get involved with the legal system for a relationship-related problem. Men may feel humiliated if they're afraid of a woman, who is usually smaller and perceived as less dangerous. Certain acts, such as raising a clenched fist, are viewed as dangerous when the aggressor is male and the target female, yet may be considered laughable when the roles are reversed.

The tendency to see female stalking or aggression as humorous can backfire, keeping men—and even boys—from getting the support they need. Jerry, a former student of mine, told me that he had been cyberstalked throughout high school by a girl he was friends with during his freshman year. His friends made fun of her obsessive Facebook posts about him and her repeated efforts to get him to chat over IM by changing her user name, which he blocked. "I joined in the laughter," he said. "I didn't want it to be awkward. I didn't want to say I was scared of this girl. Who wouldn't have laughed at me because of that?"

At one point, he was so alarmed by her behavior that he confessed his fears to a school guidance counselor. She suggested that he give a photo of the girl to school security. Confiding in the guidance counselor made him feel a little better, and the girl never showed up at his school. But looking back from the vantage point of several years, he said the school should have done more. "I was pretty lucky," he said. "She seemed unhinged. She could have brought a gun to school—and then wouldn't they [school officials] have felt bad that they didn't take me more seriously?" If he had been a girl, he said, "everyone would have pounced" on the situation. "Because I'm a boy, I'm supposed to take care of these things. But what if I couldn't?"

Jerry, in other words, didn't quite fit what Sinclair and other relationship aggression researchers call the "good victim" prototype. Submissive, frightened women and girls, for instance, are "good victims," perceived as deserving of support. Men and teenage boys, who are "supposed to take care of these things," make far less acceptable victims, particularly if they or their peers laugh about their aggressor or act in other ways unfitting to victimhood. Luke, for example, seemed to relish retelling the tantalizing bits of his "porch diver" story—how willing Dara was to bed him right away, and how, the night after the police made her leave his house, she called to ask him to see her again, "just for sex." He told me he was briefly tempted, then turned her down. "I said to myself, 'This woman dove into my concrete and tile porch, bloodied her nose, and called the police on me. This is a woman I don't want in my life.'"

This kind of swagger, says Langhinrichsen-Rohling, may be a consequence of "men's socialization scripts," which "promote the notion that they should be ready to have a sexual experience with any woman, at any time." Dara's determined pursuit at once alarmed Luke *and* gave him a pleasurable ego boost—two seemingly irreconcilable states, at least for the good victim. In a kind of macho version of slut-shaming, Luke's buddies told him that he "let himself in for it" by accepting the opportunity to sleep with Dara only hours after they met. "Any woman who's going to do that has a screw loose to begin with," they said.

Male stalking victims are viewed as more responsible for what happened to them than are female victims, according to published studies. The research also shows that female stalkers are not seen as being as much cause for concern as male stalkers. What the studies' findings amount to is an attitude akin to "rape culture" misperceptions about women. Sexual assault awareness campaigns have for years worked to debunk the idea that women are "asking" to be raped if they dress provocatively or seem to lead a man on. While these efforts haven't eliminated these beliefs, they've done a lot to raise awareness of them. Yet we haven't started to confront the ways in which, in the power dynamics of relationship pursuit, we put a similar false onus on men. We buy into the myth that their desire for sex is perpetual and undiscriminating, so there is no such thing as unwanted pursuit.

Under this myth, any refusal of a woman's advances, then, seems a lie. As writer James Lasdun put it in his memoir, *Give Me Everything You Have: On Being Stalked*, rejecting a woman's love is, in the pagan world, a "sin against nature" that is "inevitably punished." He points to the story of Hermaphroditus, who rejects the advances of the nymph Salmacis. In revenge, she wraps him in an embrace. Their two bodies merge into one, creating the first hermaphrodite. Her predatory hug possesses him and emasculates him at once.

Lasdun's saga of being cyberstalked began in 2005, when a talented former student he calls Nasreen emailed him asking for help with finding an agent for her novel. Her messages were at first professional, then flirtatious, then obsessive and hateful. She contacted his employers to disparage him as a writer and teacher. She excoriated him in the reader-review section for his novels on Amazon and other sites. She submitted racist and sexist essays from his email address to publications. She accused him of affairs with students, plagiarism, and arranging for her own rape. At one point, her cyberstalking escalated to violent threats against him and his family.

In many ways, Lasdun is a "good victim." He is a married father of two children who were in grade school when the stalking began. Though he confesses in his memoir that he privately had felt some degree of attraction to Nasreen, he clearly and immediately rejected her advances. He took seriously the vengeful response that followed. Pagan dictates aside, he told me he never felt the stalking was "an affront to my masculinity." He just wanted it to stop. Her relentlessness was taking over his life. "I was obsessed myself," he said. "I couldn't think of anything else." He went to the police and gained the support of an NYPD detective familiar with the kind of behavior Nasreen was exhibiting. But there wasn't much the detective could do beyond calling Nasreen and warning her to stop. She lived in California, and what she had done constituted only a misdemeanor. So Lasdun did what writers do: He wrote about what he was going through.

Lasdun told me that he found sexual politics a "limited" way to understand stalking. "I think, on the whole, it's more fruitful to look at stalking as a thing people do to other people," he said. "It's a human problem." Yet a good deal of the critical response to *Give Me Everything You Have* turned out to be what he called a "minefield." "There's a double standard," he said. "The amount of victim blaming surprised me."

New Yorker reviewer John Colapinto insisted that Lasdun failed to fully acknowledge his "crush" on Nasreen; rather, he "let his sexual nature get the better of him" to "accidentally (and dangerously) lead on a paranoid fantasist." Jessica Freeman-Slade of *The Millions* accused him of sounding "like Humbert Humbert, more complicit than innocent, more culpable than defensible"—as if, instead of being a stalker's target, Lasdun was a scheming molester, Nasreen no more powerful than a confused and manipulated tween. Nick Richardson of *The London Review of Books* suggested that the very act of publishing his account made Lasdun the victor against Nasreen's "digital menace," which "almost doesn't qualify as stalking" because there was no physical confrontation: "Lasdun got a book out of Nasreen, while she remains alone, her novel unpublished, clearly very ill." Jenny Turner in *The Guardian* charged Lasdun of failing to see the possibility that "Nasreen is in terrible distress"—and of approaching his story with "an almost total lack of self-irony."

Irony, it seems, is mandatory for the male target of female stalking—otherwise, we might have to acknowledge that what he's gone through is real. We'd much rather believe in the stalking woman as a symbol of resistance against the tyranny of the mentor, the indignities of sexual rejection, and the anguish of obsession. If rejecting a woman is a sin against nature, telling the story of her vengeance may not offer much redemption. It may even amplify the transgression. It's no surprise that many male targets of stalkers choose to keep quiet and try to handle the problem themselves.

MITCH, A MEDICAL anthropologist, did not dial 911 the day Anne broke in to his living room. She had been stalking him for months. They had dated briefly when they were in their twenties, after he returned home from Vietnam. He remembered her as insecure and belligerent, particularly toward women she perceived as rivals. After they broke up, she "literally vanished." He didn't see her again until he was in his fifties, married, and browsing through a sporting-goods store in a shopping mall. "Oh, look who it is," Anne said. She was a tall woman dressed in a short royal blue dress and high heels. He found her striking.

"I suppose we can pick up where we left off," she said.

"I don't think so," he said, and told her he was married.

"That can be changed," she replied curtly, and left the store.

He spotted her watching him nearly every day after. She drove past, staring right at him, while he was waiting in line to get ice cream for his nieces. She pulled up behind him in the parking lot where he was picking up his teenage son and daughter. "They could have been my kids," she said, then drove away. At a party, she walked up to him with a friend and introduced him: "This is my ex-lover, soon to be my lover again." On a beach outing, he caught sight of Anne confronting his wife as he paddled nearby on a kayak. He rushed back to shore. "When she saw me, she said, 'Oh, shit,' and drove off on her motorcycle," he said.

He and his wife went to Ukraine for six weeks. They got home around noon. Within hours, Anne telephoned. "Oh, you're back now," she said.

When he ran into her by himself in a grocery store, he asked her, "Are you threatening me?"

"You're going to find out," she said.

One day he and his wife left on a brief errand without locking their door. When they returned home, Anne was sitting in the living room. Mitch's three Rottweilers were standing guard around her. "They wouldn't let me leave," Anne said.

"What are you doing here?" Mitch asked.

"Snooping," she said calmly.

"Get out," he said.

"Don't give me orders!" she said.

Mitch bristled. "It's not an order. Just get out," he said, and she did.

He thought of calling the police to report her, but then told himself that they wouldn't do anything. After Vietnam, he said, he'd lost his trust in authority and the government. Several days later, he asked a friend in law enforcement what he could do. The friend told Mitch that so far, there were no grounds to do anything. "She broke in to my home," Mitch protested. His friend explained that because Mitch hadn't called the police then, he wouldn't be able to prove anything. Even if he could prove that she'd threatened him, all the police would do was issue an order of protection forbidding her to come within a thousand yards of him. "Those measures are ineffectual," Mitch said. "I learned in the service how to be effectual. I knew how to take care of my own problems."

He felt he could defend himself against her, but he worried about his wife and kids. He began to fantasize about blowing up her car with her in it. Then, after Anne had been stalking him for about six months, she pulled her vanishing act again. He hasn't seen her since.

In the wake of her disappearance, Mitch suffered terrible personal losses. His elderly mother died after a long illness. Eight months later, his wife, who was much younger than he was, died suddenly of a cerebral aneurysm. In his grief, he continued to feel a fierce rage at Anne. "It had an extremely personal impact on my psyche," he said. "It made me angry that someone could try to control me that way, that someone could make me feel that I was not in total control of myself."

He told me that she was one of the factors that pushed him "off the deep end" after his wife died. He went into therapy and was diagnosed with post-traumatic stress disorder, which began in his early childhood and was exacerbated by Vietnam. Anne retriggered him, he told me, and he began to realize in therapy that it was okay for him to seek help when he didn't feel in control—a realization he could not have reached while Anne was actively stalking him.

Mitch had been caught in what Langhinrichsen-Rohling calls a "double jeopardy" for male victims of stalking. If they are reluctant to show or even feel much fear, they are less likely to seek help from friends, professionals, or law enforcement. If they do seek help, they may not get much, because society doesn't take female-on-male stalking seriously.

As Mitch recognized, orders of protection have only a limited reach. Studies of orders of protection show that they are associated with a reduced risk of violence toward victims who obtain them. But a study that looked at the efficacy of orders of protection in stalking cases revealed that more than 81 percent of the orders issued for male victims are violated, along with about 69 percent of the orders issued for female victims. Lasdun found that because his cyberstalker lived in California, he had very little recourse. Orders of protection didn't apply. Much of what she did was considered aggravated harassment, a mere misdemeanor, not worth the expense of extraditing her to New York. After she threatened murder, investigators told Lasdun that an extradition could move forward. But two of his colleagues had also become targets.

They objected to the extradition after learning that once Nasreen's hearing in New York was over, she would be set free to do as she wished, in much closer proximity to them.

Lasdun's experiences reveal the risks of identifying as a victim of stalking—indeed, of any kind of bullying or harassment. You'll be subject to scrutiny and suspicion, and you might never get the protection you deserve, not to mention the justice. Mitch's saga, in turn, exposes the possible consequences of refusing the victim label and staying invisible: If you can't come to terms with your inability to control your attacker, you might implode. The very least we can do for male targets of female stalking, whether they call themselves victims or not, is to let go of our own attachment to the impossibility of their suffering, and refuse to give their pursuers the gender pass.

7

Crush

UNREQUITED LOVE AS GIRL POWER

꘎

CLARA STEPPED ONSTAGE, LEADING A troupe of nine-year-old girls dressed in iridescent purple and green costumes. They danced around the boat where the teenage girl playing Ariel, the Little Mermaid, sat fluttering her eyes and grinning at Prince Eric. "Kiss the girl," my daughter and her ensemble urged him. His kiss, as the story goes, had the power to restore the Little Mermaid's melodious voice, which she'd traded in for a pair of legs and the chance to win the prince's love.

I watched my daughter dance. Her unruly curls were pulled back. The bit of makeup I'd allowed her brought out the outlines of the young woman she would become. She loved to be onstage, loved the big colorful productions her performing arts program staged every spring.

I loved to watch them, but I had my qualms about this year's show choice. The mermaid gives up not one but two essential parts of herself—her tail and her voice—to go after a guy who couldn't even recognize her as his rescuer. The musical and Disney-film versions of the story make her sacrifice pay off. The prince returns her love, and the two live happily ever after. In the original Hans Christian Andersen version, the Little Mermaid is turned into sea foam for her troubles and evaporates into the heavens. She gains an immortal soul, which, in Hans Christian Andersen's worldview, is the ultimate spiritual reward. From another vantage point, her end looks a lot more like suicide by unrequited love.

When my daughter was a preschooler, we talked about both versions of *The Little Mermaid*. "How about that," I used to say in my Mommy-makes-a-little-fun-of-fairy-tales voice. "She gives up her beautiful voice, suffers great pain, and all for some guy who doesn't even know she exists? Not smart."

"Yeah. Duuuuh," Clara would join in. It was part of our ongoing conversations about which princesses were smart (The Paper Bag Princess, The Princess Knight, and later, Merida in *Brave* and Rapunzel in *Tangled*) and not smart (Snow White, who not only talked to a stranger when there was a death warrant out for her but also *ate that stranger's apple*).

Clara's princess phase passed years ago. She has yet to be struck by her own romantic yearnings, though she comes home with reports about classmates' crushes. A couple of girls claim they've already gone on "dates." The inevitability of these feelings in her life has been very much on my mind as I've worked on this book. How will she handle it? How will *I*? The Little Mermaid embodies a main peril of unrequited love: self-sacrifice. I remain uneasy about the prospect that one day, dreams of a prince—or, more likely, some clueless dude in her math class—might take over my daughter's lively imagination.

Through most of her childhood, she's largely tuned out boys, which is developmentally quite common. Children spend most of their time with same-sex peers. I was the same way. Boys weren't on my radar until, all at once, around sixth grade, they were. It was a shock to my system to find myself so preoccupied with Danny, a boy with feathered-back dark hair in the style of Shaun Cassidy, the pop-culture It Boy at the time. I had spoken to Danny maybe twice. I did nothing about my feelings and told no one, but my emotions must have showed. One day I found a note in my locker saying, "Will you go out with me? Love, Danny." My chest squeezed and my face grew hot, a beat before I took in the loopy handwriting, clearly a girl's penmanship. My friend had written the note to tease me.

Part of me wished my daughter could simply skip this kind of humiliation. She is so self-assured now, with a healthy aversion to being treated poorly or ignored by her peers; she has an enviable aptitude for distancing herself from classmates, male and female, who aren't decent to her. I can hardly imagine her feeling so vulnerable. My mom friends and I speak about the advent of romantic feelings in our daughters with some degree of dread, *The Little Mermaid* a cautionary tale: One day our daughters will feel as Ariel felt, pining over someone impossibly remote, distracted from school and family, and given, we fear, to sacrificing her voice. Voice—finding it, keeping it, cultivating it, using it—was the feminist metaphor for selfhood that guided us in college into our own adulthood. Crushes seem to threaten that process of becoming. And I certainly did not want my daughter to lose herself to someone the way I did.

But as I've unpacked unrequited love in these pages, I've been a steady defender of its essence. This fraught state can be a meaningful one, if we heed it carefully. Watching *The Little Mermaid* musical onstage, I was struck by one scene in particular: Ariel, surrounded by treasures salvaged from humans (including the iconic fork she uses to comb her curls), dreams of a life beyond her sheltered underwater existence. The song she sings, "Part of Your World," is about her desire to rebel against her overprotective father, the king of the sea, and be "where the people are."

In the classic structure of musical theater, "Part of Your World" is what's called the "I wish" song—when a main character declares what she wants, and this gets the story going. At this point, she is just *wishing*, the quintessential state of the adolescent girl. She wants to leave behind the constraints of childhood and transform herself into someone new. She wants to love and be loved by someone who represents these possibilities.

Ariel's story moves on to fulfill her fantasy. She wins the impossible beloved and gets back her voice. Plenty of girls with a crush don't get any further than the "I wish" song. They're not going to get the guy. But the state of wishing can be useful. Closer scrutiny of the crush suggests that this fraught state does not have to be a threat to a girl's emerging adult self. Unrequited love has the capacity to *enable* these emerging selves—as such, we may be better off viewing the crush not with trepidation but as opportunity.

THE WORD "CRUSH" originated in the nineteenth century as a description for a crowded social gathering or a dance where marriageable young men and women might jostle against each other and meet. In a time of stricter courtship protocols and gender segregation, crushes offered a chance for nearness and contact, the throngs of people offering a cover, a sense of the accidental, for the moments when sleeve brushed sleeve or shoulder bumped shoulder. Such situations likely fostered deeper longings, the hope to bump into a specific someone—what we would consider a crush now.

Today the door to that crowded Saturday-night dance of yore is, in the virtual world, perpetually open, with the digital blurt of a chat message alert or text often serving as that first spark of flirtatious contact. A teen outside of Boston told me that when she was in middle school, she jumped on her laptop every day after she got home. As she picked away at her homework, she maintained at least half a dozen chat conversations with her friends. She knew she wasn't focusing as well as she should on her assignments, but she couldn't force herself to close the IM program. "If my crush was online, I would stay to see if he would chat with me," she said. When she was in high school, the explosion of social media apps made analyzing romantic intentions even more complicated. Pressing "like" on five Instagram photos of a peer became code for being attracted to the person. Flirting and arguing took place over "subtweets"—enigmatic 140-character announcements ("I finally feel someone understands me"; "I hate being ignored") aimed at one person, yet tweeted out to hundreds of peer followers. "Relationships and crushes have gone very public in one way, and then in another way, they're under the radar because people don't show their affection as much in person," she said.

Taking seemingly private communications about yearning and disappointment into the social media thicket can serve different purposes for young people with crushes, according to Ilana Gershon, an anthropology professor at Indiana University who's often referred to as an "Internet ethnographer." In the interviews she conducted for her book, *The Breakup 2.0: Disconnecting over New Media,* she found that for some people, social media announcements about their romantic intentions and disappointments helped minimize their vulnerability. "If you're not saying it directly to a person, then you're not forcing them to own it or to respond. You're introducing a certain amount of ambiguity," she said. Other people are motivated by an opposite impulse: the need to make their feelings "as important as possible by having other people called forward as witnesses, who have to engage and respond and support you."

Historically, new communication technologies were introduced along with clear protocols for how to use them. When the telephone became available to consumers, companies hired people to monitor conversations. They even sent letters reprimanding women who talked too long. "Now we don't have anyone to tell us what's appropriate and inappropriate," Gershon said. The five-Instagram-photo-rule my teen source mentioned became flash policy for her peer group, but it may not apply elsewhere. A girl who texts with her boyfriend throughout the day thinks of what they're doing as part of an expected conversation that is *never over*," even after he has told her he needs a break from the relationship; their steady digital connection somehow doesn't figure in, even as it disrupts the distance he has said he wants. "I have a lot of sympathy for young people because they're learning how to manage what it means to love as they are learning what it means to communicate using these technologies," Gershon said. "No one has the same shared expectations."

WHILE THE DIGITAL world that stokes teen crushes may be new, the feelings underneath are not. The adolescent crush is an expected rite of passage. Since the early 1900s, psychologists have recognized the developmental validity of puppy love, teacher and camp counselor crushes, and zealous same-sex adolescent friendships (particularly among girls in single-sex schools), characterized by expressions of undying commitment, affection, and fierce jealousy; most youths, these early researchers reassured, would move on from these "homosexual attachments" as they grew older and had more exposure to the opposite sex. Today's psychological literature on crushes in childhood and adolescence continues to see the unilateral romantic fantasies of the young as stalwartly normal. Nearly every girl has had at least one crush by the age of fourteen. Girls start crushing earlier than boys because girls hit puberty sooner, a time when romantic fantasies and desires fire up. These early crushes are part of a time of transition, when kids go from virtually ignoring the opposite sex to beginning to imagine relationships with them; gay and lesbian youths start to grapple with their sexual orientation and adjust the ways they relate to same-sex peers. In early adolescence, most kids spend a lot of time fantasizing about romance and people they like, often without trying to start a relationship.

Crushes are one of the main ways younger adolescents connect to the opposite sex. They are more likely to have a crush on an acquaintance than a good friend of the opposite sex, and far more likely to have a crush than a relationship. Early dates or relationships tend to be rare, awkward, and ephemeral. Girls at this point are in what researchers call the "initiation phase" of adolescent romantic relationships. Socially, they are figuring out how they might choose and relate to prospective partners by talking a lot about them with their friends. They ponder who likes whom and how they might go about getting a crush's attention. Internally, the most detailed, vivid, and emotionally intense aspect of their nascent romantic lives is fantasy, not real interaction.

As kids move through their teens, their fantasies become more goal-oriented. A ninth-grader will probably spend more time fantasizing about a crush than an eleventh-grader, and she's more likely to keep her crush a secret. The eleventh-grader tends to see her crush as a precursor to a relationship. She'll be more overt in letting her crush know how she feels. Once she realizes he's not interested, she's more likely to move on; if he is interested, the crush may transition into a mutual relationship. This developmental pattern seems nicely utilitarian. In reality, it's not nearly so neat. Crushes can get out of hand at any age. A girl who wants to make major life decisions to include a boy who doesn't return her feelings, or a teen who cyberstalks a boy who has asked her to leave him alone, isn't engaging in anything that will benefit her.

But in general, the landscape of a teen crush is a far safer and more beneficial one than the rough terrain of early relationships and sex, particularly for younger teens. Adolescents in relationships are particularly susceptible to one another's influence. A teen partner can be a super-concentrated form of peer pressure, affecting delinquency rates, grades, and academic engagement. Though the partner's impact can be positive—she's inspired to work hard in school because he's brainy, for example—it's more likely that it won't be. Romantic relationships in high school and early adolescence are linked with lower grades and standardized test scores. Ninth-graders who date seriously or are sexually active are much less likely than their peers to graduate from high school and enroll in college. Girls involved in romantic relationships have higher rates of depression than boys in relationships and peers of both sexes who don't date at all. The more relationships that adolescents have, and the younger they are when they start them, the greater the probability they will suffer from depression. The negative effects of early romantic involvement decrease as kids move into their late teens. Teen dating can also have positive impacts, giving teens great pleasure, emotional support, and useful experience in handling intimacy and conflict. But dating relationships are their single greatest source of stress.

Crushes, in contrast, provide a kind of emotional cocoon—a place to incubate intense emotion without the level of contact and influence entailed by a mutual relationship. Richard Weissbourd, a child and family psychologist at Harvard's School of Education and the Kennedy School of Government, said that in middle school and high school, very few people are developmentally ready for the "real empathy, self-awareness, discipline, and courage" that it takes to have an intimate relationship. "Some middle school and high school students clearly have healthy romantic relationships, but a crush can be an important form of enacting something in fantasy as a way of preparing for something in reality," he said.

His words made me think of Nikki. By her junior year at her large public high school in the South Bronx, it seemed like "everyone had a boyfriend" except her. She was an only child. Her mother, who worked in an administrative job for the city, raised Nikki largely by herself; her father had been estranged from the family for years. Her mother doggedly tried to ward off the dangers of the neighborhood, one of the most troubled areas of the country, where the poverty rate was the highest in the nation. The area was rife with drugs, gangs, and girls who became mothers before they finished high school.

Nikki spent a lot of time alone. She was forbidden to hang around outside or play with the other kids in the building. Her mother was worried about their older, tougher siblings. She didn't want anything to "escalate," she explained. When Nikki was in her teens, her mother warned her more specifically about men. Her mother's own first love, the man she lost her virginity to, had betrayed her cruelly. After they'd had sex one afternoon, he let a friend into his apartment. He tried to hold Nikki's mother down so the friend could rape her. She escaped. The message to Nikki was always "be independent and don't rely on anyone."

Craig first caught Nikki's attention in honors history class, during their junior year. Craig was debating with another girl about the Jim Jones massacre. The girl insisted that Jones killed all his followers. Craig parried back that plenty of the followers were responsible for their own deaths. "They *wanted* to drink the Kool-Aid," he scoffed.

"Then I was like, 'Oh my God, he is so hot,'" Nikki said in a whisper, as if, during our interview, Craig could somehow hear her. She was impressed with how smart he sounded. She was tall and lanky, qualities that made her feel awkward, and he was tall and lanky, too. "So he can relate," she said.

She joined the senior trip committee so she would have an excuse to ask him where he thought the class should go, but she couldn't manage much conversational momentum beyond that. She rarely spoke directly to him. Her crush was characterized by a slapstick goofiness. She'd impishly peer inside the room where he had a ninth-period class. If he turned to look at her, she'd bolt away, her backpack flapping against her back. She and her girlfriends prank-called Craig's apartment, using *67 to shield her caller ID.

She created fake Myspace and Facebook accounts, using photos of girls she thought were attractive. She didn't dare friend Craig, but she friended his brother Ky. Her IM chats with Ky turned into "heavy dirty talking," with Nikki playing the role of the attractive temptress "Sarah," who casually sneaked in the occasional query about Craig. She got up the nerve to ask Ky if Craig was interested in anyone. Ky told her he was—someone who was short. She thought, "What's short?" "Some guys, if they're tall, they think five foot nine is short," she said. Then Ky said the girl his brother liked had long hair. Then Nikki knew the girl Craig was interested in definitely wasn't her.

She cried herself to sleep. She was getting nowhere. Her life seemed further and further away from the reality of her other classmates. One day a friend of hers made a joke about throwing a sex party. Nikki blurted out, "Girl, aren't you a virgin?" As soon as the words came out of her mouth, she realized that her friend probably wasn't. By asking the question, she was exposing her naïveté—and her own embarrassing lack of experience.

The summer before Nikki left for college, she got her first cell phone. One of the first things she did with it was head to Craig's apartment. She took along a male friend and sent him inside the building while she waited across the street. Her friend aimed the phone at the door of Craig's unit, 2A, and filmed it for a few seconds. Nikki wanted the video of Craig's door, which she'd never seen in person, "so I could feel like I was there, to have a memorabilia, a souvenir," she told me.

What was behind that door? The private life of a boy she was obsessed with but barely knew. The prospect of a relationship and sex—which she both wanted and had been taught to view with great trepidation. Throughout the summer after her high school graduation, she peered at the door, pixilated and shaky on her tiny cell phone screen. Even after she left for college and stopped watching the file as often, she couldn't bring herself to delete it. At the end of her freshman year, her phone broke. She couldn't salvage anything on it.

There is much that *can* be salvaged from a crush. Nikki's longing for Craig was her first experience of intense desire, with the considerable risks of consummation safely behind closed doors; there was no chance that loving Craig would interfere with her education and her future, the way boyfriends and sex did with so many of her peers. Her crush, she told me, also led her to reckon with the impact of her father's absence and her isolated upbringing. "My dad wasn't like a dad growing up," she told me. "It was just me and my mom. I was very lonely. I just wanted a friend I could talk to. I watched a lot of movies, and I think I'm influenced by a lot of love movies and love stories." Another teen described her crushes as experiences that made her stronger by helping her see that she could get over disappointment. Rejection helped her develop her "logical side." When a boy she had a crush on became interested in one of her friends, she forced herself to think through the situation. "There's nothing I can do," she told herself. "If they like each other and he is happier, why should I waste my time being sad about it? There's a world of other males out there."

Though plenty of teens nurture their crushes in secret, Weissbourd has observed that the obsessive nature of unrequited love can drive some young people to become quite voluble and expressive, even if they usually aren't that open about their feelings. Parents should seize the opportunity to connect. "It's really important just to listen to them, and think about what kind of meaning they are making from the crush, and reflect on it with them," he said. "Then ask yourself: 'How can I be a good parent for this experience?'"

Jennifer Powell-Lunder, a clinical psychologist who counsels adolescents in the New York City suburbs, said that part of good parenting means avoiding the tendency to overidentify with your daughter's crush. A mother who assures her daughter, "I know what you're going through," threatens a teen's sense of identity. "They believe no one has ever felt the way they do, because it's so intense," she said.

Carl Pickhardt, an Austin, Texas–based psychotherapist and author of several books on parenting adolescents, sees crushes as important "emotional risk taking." Parents should help their kids turn their attention away from whether the crush likes them back and toward themselves, particularly if the target of the crush is someone who isn't likely to return their feelings. What does their crush tell them about what they value in a person? Are those values meaningful or superficial? What can teens learn about themselves that might help them in future relationships? "If you can get that data out of them, you can refer it back to them," Pickhardt said. "These qualities describe the other person, but it also describes your child and what matters to her." The crush, then, becomes a kind of attenuated dress rehearsal, a way to practice for the real thing in the relative safety of a girl's own head.

DURING MARISSA'S SENIOR year at an all-girls' Catholic high school in suburban Buffalo, she fell hard for a physics teacher. He was in his twenties and new on the faculty that year. She didn't have his class and saw him mainly in the lunchroom when he was on duty as a monitor. "Everyone thought he was cute at first, and then when they got to know him, they thought he was weird," she said. "My experience was different, though. I didn't get over him."

It was precisely his weirdness that Marissa liked. She was interested in science and planned to study physical anthropology and osteology—"bones and such"—in college. She had always been very shy, and she didn't have much contact with boys. She had never been in a relationship. After three years of not caring much about how she looked when she went to school, she started wearing makeup and primping. At lunch, "I'd become more outgoing," she said. "I wanted him to notice me and want to get to know me."

One day she got up the nerve to ask him a question about chaos theory. He answered her and told her he was impressed with her query. From that point on, she felt more comfortable around him. It was the start of what she calls their "relationship in quotes"—

because it was "hardly a relationship, certainly not a romantic one." She daydreamed about him constantly, her mind wandering in class. She'd think she see him looking at her in the lunchroom, then she'd chastise herself for being so stupid. "There was definitely an internal struggle happening in my head for several months, going back and forth between how perfect we'd be together and how stupid and foolish I was being about the whole thing," she said. "But no matter how much I tried to talk myself down, I could not stop thinking about him. School, work, while I was driving, before I fell asleep at night."

The developments of her crush on the teacher shaped her senior year. One day at lunch she and her friends were goofing around in front of her new laptop, taking pictures of themselves. She invited the teacher to join them, and he did, giving her images that she would return to again and again. At the end of the school year, she went to a school-sponsored party after the prom and spent most of the night talking to him. "I was in heaven," she said. Her date, a male friend, asked if she had a crush on her teacher. "I said, 'No comment.' I figured it was so obvious, there was no point in lying."

At graduation, she introduced the teacher to her parents, who invited him to stop by their house. "I was mortified. I had no idea why they would do such a thing," she said. "Then my whole family walked away, leaving me waiting for the response. There was a really long, awkward silence, and then we both said goodbye and went our separate ways."

On an innocent level, each stage of her crush echoed a "real" relationship. Marissa and the teacher connected over common interests. She became preoccupied, as do many people newly in love. The pair posed for photos. They spent an evening together at the after-prom party. She introduced him to her parents, who invited him into the fold. She fully understood that her love would always be unrequited and why she was so wrapped up in him. "It's like me trying to tell myself I want this," she told me. "But I'm still too scared to go for it in real life. It's a safe way to have these feelings without being rejected. Coming out of it I feel like I've gone through an experience in which nothing happened, but I feel like something happened. It's a process that's building up to me being ready to have a relationship."

What stood out about Marissa's experience was why she admired him—he taught science. His "weirdness" embodied for her what being into science meant. It was a kind of outsider status in the universe of her high school. The first turning point of her crush—daring to ask a smart question—connected her to that outside world. What Marissa went through is what Pickhardt would call an "identity crush": unrequited love for someone who embodies what an adolescent wants to become. It's the impulse at the heart of the status-leaping crushes on popular peers, authority figures, or celebrities. "Girl crushes" in the tween and teen years can be a tug toward lesbian sexuality, or a desire to be like the female beloved, or both. "Crushes are less an expression of the other person than they are an expression of self," Pickhardt said. "You are projecting characteristics onto the person that you find powerfully attractive."

The idea of identity crushes evoked the Jungian impulse described to me by several of my adult interview subjects: *I want this person because I want to be like him.* I thought of my own first experience of puppy love, for a boy named David whom I met at summer camp in Maine. I wrote to him often, far more than he wrote me. He lived on the Upper West Side of Manhattan, near the renowned food bazaar Zabar's, which sounded wonderfully exotic. At fourteen, he had an intellectual and cultural voraciousness that impressed me. He was a huge fan of Sting, and the literary references in the lyrics led David to read Paul Bowles and Goethe.

He saw a therapist and tossed off sophisticated phrases like "Freud would have a holiday with that one." His father managed the career of a famous violinist. After I got a letter from David or spoke with him on the phone, I'd feel piercing envy. I was a dentist's daughter in a small town so dull that kids gathered in the Grand Union parking lot for fun on Saturday nights. I went to the library and brought home a stack of books. My brother saw them on the kitchen counter. "Dream interpretation? Existentialism? Who does she think she is?" he scoffed.

My brother was on to something. I *did* want to be someone else. My desire for the boy from camp was entwined with a desire not to be subsumed by the boredom and smallness of exurban adolescence. My infatuation with him made me feel my life had taken a wrong turn. As a young girl, I'd been an avid reader and an involved student. In middle school, I began to spend hours gossiping on the telephone with friends and cared a lot less about my schoolwork. The specter of David (and he did seem to be a specter, as I dreamed about him often) made me want to be cultured and aware, to live in the world as he did. His obliviousness ended up hurting me terribly, but my feelings for him pushed me toward becoming someone I needed to be.

CRUSHES SEEM LIKE they are about giving in, the self being subsumed—crushed—by yearning. But the identity-building aspect of crushes can turn them into expressions of power and resistance. Writer Barbara Ehrenreich heard the shrieks of Beatles-obsessed tweens and teens in the mid-1960s as the first stirrings of the sexual revolution. "It was rebellious . . . to lay claim to sexual feelings. It was even more rebellious to lay claim to the *active*, desiring side of a sexual attraction: the Beatles were the objects; the girls were their pursuers," she wrote in a 1992 essay on

Beatlemania. In this light, "crush" becomes an active verb, something girls *do*; they crush standards, social ideals, their own former notions of themselves.

A similar impulse of re-creation lies behind the teen crushes enacted online today, though teens' meme-sharing and digitized quips don't have the physical intensity of Beatlemania's girl-packs. The crush has long been one of the guiding conceits of social media, as attested by the lore surrounding the horny geek founders of Facebook; they created a platform for college students to look all they wanted at their classmate crushes without anyone else having to know. As social media evolves, the looking is less undercover and more of an online performance. "Crush," "girl crush," "obsession," and other terms of longing pop up frequently in tweets, blog titles, and hashtags, along with "fangirl" and "fandom." Crushes are cool. Canadian film student Meghan Harper, in a blog essay that went viral called "Why I F**ing Love Teenage Girls," defends the celebrity crush, often dissed as annoying or frivolous. A crush on a boy-band star allows a teenage girl to "develop her sexuality in a safe environment she can control." It's love without being felt up by a boy when she's not sure she wants to be, or being pressured to text him naked pictures of herself, which might later be used to humiliate her. Celebrity crushes are a form of what social scientists, since the rise of television, have called "parasocial interaction": one-sided intimacy, at a distance, with someone famous. However compelling the fantasy, there's no significant obligation or responsibility.

Fangirls are fiercely protective of the integrity of these fantasies *as* fantasies—desire without real-life interaction or consequences. A subculture of fangirls shuns mainstream pop stars such as Justin Bieber in favor of nerdy sensitive-guy alternative celebrities who sing goofy love songs (lyrics include lines such as "if you love me / then I'll never play Halo again") on YouTube. "These guys seem nonthreatening, like a best friend, but they still have that wow factor," said Katie Speller, who runs Feminist Fiction, a Tumblr blog about feminism and fandom culture. When several underage fangirls blogged on Tumblr about being sexually exploited by YouTube performers they'd corresponded with or met in person, the online outrage built quickly and powerfully. One YouTube performer lost his record contract over allegations that he'd had sex with an underage fan; another posted a lamenting apology about his abusive relationship with an admirer. YouTube celebrity Michael Lombardo was convicted on child porn charges and jailed for manipulating underage girls into sending him sexually explicit photos and videos. Speller said that throughout these incidents, fangirls, along with outspoken female YouTube stars, "really looked out for each other. They reached out and shared their experiences and told each other they should not be forgotten and they should not be walked over."

What was threatened, Speller said, was the fangirl ethos—the liberating feeling of "unironically putting yourself into loving something." On Tumblr and Twitter, what you love and what you long for are of primary importance to teen users. Unlike Facebook, where detailed profile information is the norm, Tumblr and Twitter users often work on a first-name, pseudonym, or unnamed basis, with a vague bit of "about" information: "I like nature. I wish I was a bird." It's often impossible to tell where the user lives, how old she is, what she does when she's not online. But you'll find out plenty about what she *wants*, her blog or Twitter feed creating a digital ladder of desire. On social media, she is what she crushes on. She creates herself through the things that give her "the feels," Internet slang for an intense emotional reaction to something you come across online. The feels can come from a new paparazzi photo of Kristen Stewart or a cool pair of muddied boots. They can come from a couple embracing on a bed, from the rain outside the window falling in the jerky, repetitive fashion of GIF animation.

Then there are the digital packs of girls who get the feels from killers. They curate high school yearbook photos of Dylan Klebold and Eric Harris, mug shots of Ted Bundy, and black-and-white GIFs of teen commandos firing machine guns. They call themselves "Columbiners" and "Holmies" (after Aurora, Colorado, movie shooter James Holmes). They express their yearning in Photoshopped captions in the style of inspirational bedroom posters: "I wish I could go back in time and have a serious relationship with dylan and when things got too hard i could sit in his lap while we cried into each other," reads one Columbiner post. On Twitter, a chorus of #freejahar tweets gushes about how cute the alleged nineteen-year-old Boston Bomber, Dzhokhar Tsarnaev, is—too cute and too relatable as a young college student to do harm, some say.

Dark-side crushes are rarely about connecting to the object of yearning; in many cases, he's dead. The impossibility of the bad-guy fantasy relationship makes it "psychically comfortable" for some teens, says Jill Weber, a clinical psychologist in the Washington, D.C., area. "They project on to that person whatever they want, or things they want to feel within themselves." The creative range, irony, and oddball whimsy of teen expressions of killer crushes (one post gushes about how dreamy it would be to eat gourmet chocolates with Jeffrey Dahmer) indicate they are more about power, identity, and experimentation than a genuine desire to have a relationship. In a much discussed essay in *The Awl*, writer Rachel Monroe sees a Beatlemania-like fervor in these dark-side posts and tweets, a push back against the manufactured conventions of teen sexuality. My impression is that the rebellion is really against a far more intractable reality: the girls' own vulnerability, not only to the emotional challenge of love and sex but also to the existential challenge of living in a world of oppression and evil. If you can snuggle up to a killer, you can weaken his menace.

FOR MOST TEEN girls, the real challenge of a crush is about dealing with the force of her emotions for a boy she knows, not a killer or a pop idol. It's hard for a girl—as it can be for an adult woman—to see beyond the present tense of a crush, to grasp the possibility of an opportunity for growth until she's gotten over her feelings. Meanwhile, her life is characterized by intense vulnerability. Even if the boy hasn't been unkind to her, the fact that he doesn't love her back hurts, and she may feel a lesser person because of it. What is valued, all around her at school and in the culture at large, is relationship *success*, and she's not achieving it.

Suzi Yoonessi, a thirty-five-year-old filmmaker in Los Angeles, has vivid memories of heartbreak as a girl growing up in Buffalo in the 1990s. "It was an experience that happened over and over again," she said. "Everything is amplified when you're young because you haven't been numbed." She confided her crushes and breakups in her "epic collection" of diaries, addressing the entries to "Lemon Lima," her imaginary friend.

Yoonessi grew up listening to her Persian grandmother's fairy tales about little girls and creatures who triumphed over difficult circumstances. For her first feature film, *Dear Lemon Lima*, she wanted to create a fairy tale about lost love that captured the poignancy of the experience and gave girls a glimpse of a self-affirming future beyond. "You hear so much about girls as victims, but not of how they come back from that experience and how heartbreak can make them stronger and more empowered," she said.

Dear Lemon Lima was produced with an unabashed sugar-coated aesthetic, with bright pastel colors and curlicue-script diary entries, each "i" dotted with a heart. Set in rural Alaska, the film tells the story of thirteen-year-old Vanessa Lemor as she recovers from her breakup with Philip. He is white, entitled, and arrogant. She is the daughter of a single white mother and an Eskimo father she hasn't seen in years. Vanessa attends Philip's school on a scholarship for Native Alaskans, even though she feels estranged from her heritage. She becomes so insecure and needy about Philip that her mother, frustrated, chastises her: "How can you love anyone when you don't love yourself?" The turning point in the movie comes when Vanessa and Philip are pitted against each other as rival team captains in their school's annual Snowstorm Survivor competition. Vanessa finally sees Philip for the social climber he is. She bonds closely with her teammates, a group of fellow outcasts. To everyone's surprise, Vanessa's underdog team wins.

The movie wasn't distributed far beyond the film-festival circuit in the U.S., though I wish it had the traction of the *Twilight* series. Vanessa's triumph is the perfect antidote to Bella Swan's willingness to destroy herself over her love for a handsome vampire. I watched *Dear Lemon Lima* with Clara, as part of the not so subtle unrequited love awareness campaign I've been conducting ever since our princess-phase discussions. That probably sounds hypervigilant, but it's actually been a lot of fun. Clara still thinks romance is icky and covers her eyes when movie characters kiss. She doesn't *want* to watch the mythical happy ending of the unrequited love script, when the girl finally gets the guy or vice versa. It was much more satisfying for Clara to cheer Vanessa on to victory and proclaim that Philip was "a real idiot." I can only hope that the film has some impact on her sense of possibility later on, when she no longer finds kissing a repulsive prospect. I do realize that movies don't work medicinally. And I know that the recovery process of most real-life teen heartbreak won't be as resoundingly triumphant as Vanessa's experience. But the smaller, authentic victories over heartache can matter quite a lot.

SALLY WAS A freshman at her large southern Arizona high school when her crush on Roger, a boy in one of her classes, began. As a Mormon, she wasn't allowed to date until she was sixteen, then over a year away. Because of this rule, she took longer than her peers to get interested in boys. As her classmates started to have crushes in junior high, she remained studious and uninterested.

After Roger gave an "about me" presentation for a class they were in together, she decided to try to talk to him. "I was shy and didn't have a lot of guy friends," she said. "I decided I would have one for once. I had never had a conversation go so well. I was smooth and funny. It was kind of magical."

For the next two years, she was preoccupied with finding opportunities to get closer to Roger. She went with her friends to his soccer games. She tried to text and Facebook him, but he was antisocial online and didn't respond. She borrowed his Harry Potter books one by one. Each time she finished a book, she would return it to him and try to say something interesting about it, but she couldn't manage to get much of a conversation going. She kept trying to recapture the magic of the first time they talked, but it didn't happen. He never made the effort to talk to her first, so she soon realized he wasn't interested. "For the longest time, I was really sad about it," she said. "I was still very attached to him in this puppy-dog way. I was so upset."

Sally's mother consoled her when she needed to cry and vent. Her mother told me that she knew her daughter was in the spotlight at school. Sally had confided in so many friends that the word had spread about her crush. "He was into sports and didn't get girls," her mother said. "Everyone knew she was infatuated with him. It probably scared the shorts off of him."

I admired Sally's mother for her matter-of-fact approach to her daughter's crush, and for her humor. She joked that there were times when she wanted to "go out and beat Roger with a pan" for his obliviousness. I recognized what was behind her kidding—the feeling that you would do anything to protect your kid from the pain of not being loved. All she could do, though, was focus on her daughter's state of mind. "My goal was to walk her through it and keep her self-esteem high," she said. "I told her it happens to every-one, and it's not a reflection on her."

Sally sought creative outlets for what she was feeling. She wrote poetry and song lyrics. She got a lot more involved in her school's active theater program. "The experience exposed me to this whole new aspect of being human and feeling emotion, and I could put that into my acting," she said. Midway through her junior year, she learned that Roger was dating someone else, and she resolved to move on. Then she was cast as the outspoken lesbian feminist Enid Hoopes in the musical *Legally Blonde*, itself a fable about turn-ing romantic rejection into empowerment. Enid is a classmate and eventual friend to Elle, the show's lovelorn-girlie-blonde-turned-powerhouse-law-student protagonist. "Enid is a strong character who doesn't need a man," Sally said. "People laughed at things she believed in and had a lot of emotions about. She gets hurt, but she's able to move past it and laugh back at them. As I was playing that character, I was able to look at all the growth I did. I had been de-pendent on this one person for my happiness, and I wasn't going to be that way anymore."

As I thought about Sally's story, the prospect of coping with

Clara's first crushes no longer seemed so trying. The pain of a crush like Sally's is not something a mother looks forward to. But I could imagine looking forward to the changes that could occur after that pain subsides: a new resilience, a new repertoire of feeling—qualities my daughter can use, on the stage she cherishes or off.

8

Primal Teacher

THE TRANSFORMATIONAL POWER
OF UNREQUITED LOVE

꙳

WHEN RINA, AN OPERA SINGER, WAS A conservatory student, she fell in love with a young conductor, a rising star who would become world-renowned. What he brought to her was a rare glimpse into "something much bigger" than what she'd experienced thus far—the feeling of what the real world of professional opera was like. She spent as much time as she could in his orbit, absorbing everything he had to say about music. Even though she knew he was gay, she let herself hope that she could cultivate the deep connection she felt into some kind of transcendent, "union of the soul" relationship. Yet he held himself apart from her and the many students he entranced. "The overriding feeling I had about him was that he was never a very genuine person," said Rina, forty-three. "He was always on. Once in a blue moon, I felt like I got a piece of him when he was being honest with me."

Rina shaped her days around finding opportunities to be with the young conductor. On her way to the practice rooms, she would check the papered-over window on his office door to see if a light was glowing inside. She looked forward with childlike excitement to rehearsals with him. She felt helpless to her attraction: "I thought, 'Can I please stop feeling this way,' because I felt like a live wire the electric company had yet to shut down."

During her last semester, the conductor chose Rina for the challenging lead role in Puccini's *Suor Angelica.* The opera is about a nun whose out-of-wedlock baby was taken from her seven years before. When she learns her son has died, she is grief-stricken and swallows poison. Then she realizes she has committed a mortal sin and is destined for hell. She calls out to the Virgin Mary, pleading for absolution.

On opening night, as Rina sang this passage, she felt overcome with emotion. Her vocal cords tightened, and she wasn't experienced enough to work around it. *O Madonna, salvami!** she sang, her voice cracking "in an ugly, tense way" on the high B. She was terrified she wouldn't be able to make it through the demanding passage ahead. Then the conductor gave her "the most intense look" Rina had ever seen. "He was willing me with his eyes to get me back on track and finish the song. He knew I knew how to do it, and he was going to push me over the top," she said. "I was utterly overwhelmed."

* Oh, Madonna, save me!

Moments later, the nun realizes she is saved and is carried up to heaven. Rina's final vocal gesture was a "colossal, fortissimo high C, which came out of me gloriously by means I couldn't explain," she remembered.

It was a larger-than-life moment: the potboiler tragic love story onstage; the pivotal high note; the conductor's glare evoking Svengali, the impresario who hypnotizes a tone-deaf Trilby into becoming an opera star. Rina's triumphant finish redeemed her from her mistake, as her nun character was redeemed from her sin.

The final high note signified another kind of redemption: from the failure of unrequited love. True, the conductor would never love her back. In this respect, Rina's compulsive rounds of the conservatory and all her daydreaming were fruitless. But her obsession was also what unleashed her into a moment of transcendence and heightened her understanding of what it meant to be a performer.

Throughout her obsession with the conductor, the specter of the out-of-control stalker haunted Rina. She did everything she could to avoid making her attraction known. "I would rather die than seem to be stalking," she said. Instead, she brought "the compulsion of a stalker" to her education, harnessing the unwanted woman's blend of abjection and aggression in the service of her music. She submitted completely to the conductor's guidance. "That's an unhealthy way to be in real life," she said. "But onstage, there's an inherent sort of slave mind/slave master thing going on."

Under his direction, she could be her "purest self—really an *unself*," completely absorbed in making music. The state as she described it sounded a lot like the perfect union she'd fantasized about having with the conductor—yet she experienced it with her singing instead of with him.

We have seen how a conscious scrutiny of unrequited love can tell us a lot about what we want in our lives. We also know that if we chase unrequited love too hard, we can cause harm—to others, or ourselves, or both. Rina's story raises another important possibility: that we may be able to *do something* with unrequited love and use it to our benefit. About a third of the women in my online survey responded that their unrequited love experience "changed my life for the better." The beloved can become a taskmaster and a muse, our impossible desire for him a primal teacher, guiding us toward accomplishment and transforming our lives.

THE SEEMINGLY CONTRADICTORY outcomes of romantic obsession—constructive and hurtful—are not mutually exclusive. Rina's accomplishment did not erase the pain of the conductor's lack of interest, which she felt acutely for years, every time their paths crossed in the music world. Ancient Greeks believed the god of Eros was created out of these disparate forces. He was the offspring of Aphrodite, the goddess of beauty, and Ares, the god of war. Eros embodied the creative and destructive power of love in the figure of a mischievous child who struck lovers and poets with the "divine madness" of romantic obsession. The same kind of energy, the myth suggests, lies behind both the urge to create and the urge to love. Sappho, the ancient Greek poet whose work expresses the intensity of romantic longing, called Eros "bittersweet" for the combination of pleasurable and painful feelings his victims endured. Jungian analyst Jacqueline Wright wrote that desire, which "engages every lover in an activity of the imagination," opens up possibility because "the lover is forced to notice what is missing." This realization has the potential to make us dream, change, and create. "The creative urge that is channeled toward another person can be taken back and owned," she said.

This state, both grandiose and needy, can be highly fragile, as Sappho's own story attests. A main preoccupation of her poetry, which survives mainly in enigmatic verse fragments, is the Socratic idea of *pothos*, translated as yearning, longing, or regret for "that which is elsewhere." At times addressed to female beloveds and at times to male, her poetry moves from soaring, hopeful imagery to descriptions of great pain. The persona of Fragment 31 describes how the laughter of a beloved "puts the heart in my chest on wings." A few lines later, the sight of the same beloved leads to a mortal fit: "cold sweat holds me and shaking / grips me all, greener than grass / I am and dead—or almost / I seem to me." As poetic legend has it, Sappho ended her own life in the throes of unrequited love. She supposedly jumped off the Leucadian cliffs into the sea after Phaon, a young ferryman, rejected her. The leap, which Ovid wrote about in the *Heroides*, cannot be proved as fact. But the staying power of the story points to our fears about the creative potential of romantic obsession—that it is a precursor to ruin.

Yet accomplishment is often what rescues the unwanted woman from ruin and gives her an outlet for her restless longing. One reason why people love someone who doesn't love them back is so they can be inspired by love. Psychologists Arthur and Elaine Aron call this the "Don Quixote situation." In Miguel de Cervantes's early-seventeenth-century novel, Don Quixote devotes his chivalric quests to his unrequited love, a neighboring farm girl he renames Dulcinea. Even though she never responds, his adoration allows him to experience heightened emotion, focus his life goals, and enjoy being inspired to act heroically in someone else's name. For those in the Don Quixote situation, love is an adventure, a mystery to be solved. They are the stars of the story, privileged figures in an exciting world of emotional extremes.

Interestingly, Cervantes portrayed Don Quixote as a satirical, largely ineffectual figure. He attacks windmills, believing them to be giants, and insists on rescuing a lady from a band of what he perceives as malevolent wizards, who are in fact a group of friars. His heroism often verges on buffoonery. Better evidence of the power of being in unrequited love comes from Mary Wollstonecraft, one of the most prominent figures in the history of feminism and the author of *A Vindication of the Rights of Woman.*

In 1793, Wollstonecraft fell in love with Gilbert Imlay, a restless American entrepreneur. The first few months of their affair were idyllic. Neither lover approved of the institution of marriage and its artificial demands. Commitments, they believed, should last only as long as the feeling of love. Yet she came to believe that what they had together was sacred unto itself, creating a connection more durable than the marital bond. Imlay had a different take on the situation, which became acutely apparent after they conceived a child together. Imlay was away on business for a good deal of her pregnancy. When the baby was just a few months old, Imlay departed again, this time for London. He promised to send for Wollstonecraft and baby Fanny, who remained behind in France. He was cooling on the relationship, though, and started up with another lover. His letters to her became shorter and less frequent. She wrote to him often and with great fervor, trying to convince him of his obligation to continue to love her. He finally asked her to come to London—but not as his partner. He arranged for her to live in separate furnished lodgings. Soon after she arrived, she tried to kill herself by swallowing laudanum.

After she recovered, Imlay made a startling proposal. He asked her to travel to Scandinavia to negotiate compensation for a cargo of silver he believed had been stolen. The suggestion, in the wake of his betrayal and abandonment, was quite an audacious brush-off. He was asking his emotionally fragile ex to sally forth, baby daughter and maid in tow, on a rough and dangerous journey into unsettled territory—all for the sake of his business interests, his perennial excuse for distancing himself from Wollstonecraft. She regularly accused him of neglecting her in favor of his many commercial ventures: "You seem to be got into a whirl of projects and schemes, which are drawing you into a gulph, that, if it does not absorb your happiness, will infallibly destroy mine," she wrote from Paris in 1795. Yet there Imlay was, conspiring to draw her into that same gulph—likely hoping that it would distract her and get her out of his hair. The plan included sending her away with a sworn statement that she was his wife. The document would give Wollstonecraft the authority to act on Imlay's behalf, but it also underscored the ways he was using her. Though their transcendent union was in tatters, he didn't hesitate to give her the title of wife when it might strategically benefit him.

Wollstonecraft saw opportunity instead of insult. The mission gave her a new challenge. Even though she was working on Imlay's behalf, she was also doing what she was best at: breaking new ground as a woman. She reveled in the continual surprise of being a woman in the male role of hero-adventurer, babe in arms and all. Her journey gave her a new subject to write about. In journal entries and letters, she took in the craggy beauty of Scandinavia and brought to bear her keen analytical mind in observations of local politics and customs. She bathed in the sea, took long walks, and rode horses. She negotiated strenuously on Imlay's behalf, though she failed to get the money he sought. She was by no means cured of her obsession with him. Her letters to Imlay continued to refer to her brokenhearted state. She still struggled with thoughts of suicide and was haunted by the question of whether she and Imlay would reconcile when she returned. But a steady sense of purpose on her travels kept her from dwelling too long on sadness.

Far away from her beloved, Wollstonecraft could do something with her love. She could be someone new, even with her heavy heart. In Imlay's presence, she had to face the fact of his rejection. Once she returned to England, she discovered he had taken up with yet another lover. She tried to kill herself again. This time, she dressed in heavy velvets, weighted her pockets with rocks, and, hoping to sink quickly, jumped off the Putney Bridge into the Thames. After she was rescued, she made a few more desperate pleas for reconciliation. When she was refused again by Imlay, her thoughts returned to the adventure that had revived her spirits before. She knew her journey and the devotion that had inspired it were worth something, emotionally, creatively, and financially. She asked Imlay to return the letters she sent from Scandinavia and published many of them, enriched by her journal entries, as *Letters Written During a Short Residence in Sweden, Norway, and Denmark*.

The book was a hybrid of epistolary travelogue, memoir, political analysis, and sociology. It was a tremendous commercial success. Much of its appeal came from its subplot of longing. Her letters regularly allude, somewhat obliquely, to her heartache, often followed by reassurances that she was overcoming the pain. By the time *Letters* was published, her personal story was no secret. Instead of letting her intimations of subjugation and woe discredit Wollstonecraft's feminism (as some modern critics have done), her readers connected with the "creature of feeling and imagination" behind the astute philosopher.

Wollstonecraft was caught up in a passion that drove her to great lengths. Her letters to Imlay were compulsively frequent, her rhetoric at times as well honed as anything in *A Vindication*, at times verging on humiliating supplication: "You could restore me to life and hope, and the satisfaction you would feel, would amply repay you . . . for God's sake, keep me no longer in suspense!—Let me see you once more!" She infamously begged to be included in a ménage à trois household with him and his new lover (and that was not the first time she'd made such a proposal—she'd thrown out the idea at a previous lover, a married artist). But she fought despair by making something out of the frenzied energy of unrequited love. She cloaked herself, Don Quixote–style, in the mantle of the aspiring lover and went on a heroic journey. And the Imlay she imagined—the man with whom she shared a transcendent and enduring bond, above any social custom or law—was, like Dulcinea, a fantasy.

What she created out of the idea of him *was* real. *Letters*, the last book Wollstonecraft published, isn't her best-known work. But it contains the statement that best explains the tie between her life story and her political analysis: "We reason deeply, when we forcibly feel." Her writing was a way of turning degradation into power, of getting the last and most enduring word out of a situation that might have silenced her forever.

This gesture—of using unrequited love as a goad to creativity—has endless variations. Literary critics believe that Charlotte Brontë's impassioned letters to Constantin Héger, the married Belgian teacher with whom she was enamored, were "close to an imaginative act," her way of beginning to enact the passionate expressiveness that would distinguish *Jane Eyre* and *Villette*. Shortly after she wrote her last letter to Héger, she hatched her famous plot to publish a volume of poetry she wrote with her sisters, Anne and Emily, under the male pseudonyms Currer, Ellis, and Acton Bell. Two years later, she published *Jane Eyre*, a book that stunned its original audience with its emotional frankness.

That frankness becomes playfully raw in contemporary French conceptual artist Sophie Calle's installation, *Prenez soin de vous (Take Care of Yourself)*. She incorporated the filmed and photographed responses of more than a hundred women to a breakup email she received from her lover. She selected the women for their wide range of professional and intellectual perspectives. A criminologist pronounces her ex "an authentic manipulator" who is "psychologically dangerous"; a human rights specialist tells Calle she should be relieved to be rid of him. A woman in a short, strapless yellow dress, her straight brown hair swaying over her face like a curtain, performs a plodding conceptual dance. A nine-year-old girl wonders why, if the email author says he loves Calle, is he leaving her?

The abundance of the installation reflects the excessiveness of obsession, the endless pondering of what a lover and his rejection *means*. It is also a kind of extravagant revenge: *If you don't want me, I will make something out of us anyway.* This threat comes from within the relative safety of art. Chris Kraus's 1997 novel *I Love Dick* is part one-sided epistolary novel, part confessional diary, and part public document of her real-life exhaustive and failed obsession with the eponymous Dick, a British cultural critic teaching at a university in California. He responds to her outpourings mainly with silence, evasion, and a single night in his bed; when she asks him to have sex with her, he consents with the evasive "I'm not uncomfortable with that idea." She has said that the real Dick was so alarmed by the publication of the novel that he was going to sue her for invasion of privacy, then changed his mind.

There are less edgy expressions of unrequited longing pretty much everywhere. At any given moment, you can find an unwanted woman who makes art out of lost love at an open-mike night, or in a community poetry workshop, or in the Top 40 rotation on the radio.

WE HAVE FAMILIAR ways of describing what happens when people make use of frustrated love. There's the Freudian idea of sublimation, the deflecting of sexual desire into higher pursuits. We may simply say the unwanted woman has finally found the right distraction, following the "Stay busy!" admonition so common in women's magazine articles about Getting Over Him. Yet these explanations don't really take into account the *devotional* aspect of what unrequited love can inspire. Wollstonecraft traveled and wrote not in spite of Imlay, not to forget Imlay, but because of Imlay. In her precarious state, if she could not see these pursuits as being for him, she probably would not have taken them on. Kraus has said that Dick "gave me someone to write to," the mystery of his silence impelling her work.

What is it about the state of romantic obsession that induces some unrequited lovers to action and creation? Semir Zeki, a professor of neuroaesthetics at University College London and a pioneer in the modern study of visual perception, asserts that creativity is a fundamental human response to the frustrations of love. We carry within us an inherited universal ideal of passionate love as an experience of union; love stories, mythology, and philosophy from both Western and non-Western cultures portray the desire of two lovers to merge into one being. The neurochemistry of passionate love makes us feel that this ideal is within our grasp. The release of dopamine in the reward center of the brain causes euphoria and exhilaration. Activity in the amygdala, where the fear response is generated, quiets down, promoting feelings of bravery. There's less blood flow to areas of the brain associated with judgment and negative emotions. The self, so emboldened and accepting, is readied to give itself over, as these changes in the brain weaken the divide between self and other, reinforcing the concept of union in love.

But a true merging exists only as an imagined ideal. Human experience will always fall short. Even in a loving sexual relationship, partners are confined to their separate selves. Several recent studies indicate that the release of dopamine is as connected to desire—the expectation of reward—as it is to the feeling of receiving the rewards of love and sex. The reward of physical and emotional intimacy leads to longing for more. The climax, as Zeki puts it, immediately becomes an anticlimax.

The impossibility of fully experiencing romantic oneness with another gives the unrequited lover a strange advantage when it comes to creativity. "Be gone from me! Love for you so engages me that I have no time for you," Majnun reprimands his beloved, Layla, in the renowned Persian fable. Her presence disrupts his created fantasy of their perfect love, expressed through the poetry he writes in the sand. He can invest all he wants in his creation; it draws him closer to the ideal than Layla—who was married off to another—ever could.

Creativity, as Zeki puts it, is a way of coping with the melancholy of unsatisfied yearning for unity. Creativity can step in as a way to respond to the gap between the "unity in love" concept and reality. Creative effort—exerted by the business manager, the child building a sand castle, the painter, the poet—engages the brain in a struggle similar to the struggle to love. Both involve the reward system, the brain's quest for satisfaction. Both the lover and the artist have the challenge of creating something real out of a concept in their heads. Both will, more often than not, find that reality falls short. Both will try again and again to figure out how to "get it right." Just as I once strategized and restrategized ways into B.'s heart—coy distance and waiting? insistent confrontation?—I will rewrite this paragraph many times.

The magnitude of feeling varies, of course; my diligence in crafting this paragraph is only a quiet echo of my diligence in the pursuit of B. But the fundamental similarities in the processes of creativity and passionate love matter. They are both a form of emotional currency. We ponder to what extent one pursuit can be exchanged for another. Hence our long-standing intrigue with the virgin authoress, a stock figure of nineteenth-century literary history. She makes herself a nun in the Church of Art, living her life without mutual romantic love. The shadow of unrequited love frequently hangs over her, creating mysteries: Who was the man behind Jane Austen's insights into romance—Tom Lefroy or Dr. Samuel Blackall? Who gave rise to Emily Dickinson's heartsick verse—Reverend Charles Wadsworth, her mentor and correspondent? Her sister-in-law, Susan Gilbert?

These spinsters seem to have made a bargain with Eros: Strike me with your arrow, and I will make art instead of love. This sort of deal frees them to dwell on the imagined perfection of ideal love instead of mutual love's faulty lived reality. In this way they are like Dante and Werther, yet the spinster artist has even more at stake. Mutual love almost inevitably led to domesticity, and babies, and far less time and space for a creative mind. The unwanted woman, historically, was a freer woman. We still contend with this legacy. The pop singer Adele wrote the Grammy-award winning "Someone Like You" and the rest of her smash-hit album *21* in response to the end of a "rubbish relationship." When she fell in love again and got pregnant, she offered a satisfying resolution to her woe. One of my daughter's friends, at age nine, proclaimed exuberantly: "Adele has a new boyfriend and she's going to have a baby and she'll never be sad again!" (Her mother sagely warned her that life has no such guarantees.) There was one immediate drawback to Adele's happy ending: less of her music. Adele announced that she would need to take a break from touring for several years—leaning out, we might call it—to help her new domesticity survive. "If I am constantly working, my relationships fail," she said.

The misery of imperfect love, Zeki writes, "generates splendors in its turn" with the brain's capacity to "turn that discontent into creative achievement." Based on existing brain scan research on how people respond to art, Zeki surmised that the creative process likely involves the orbital-frontal cortex, thought to be related to emotion and reward in decision-making. As the brain lights on a work of art that it considers beautiful, blood flow steps up in this area, causing a feeling of satisfaction; a decrease in blood flow is a sign of dissatisfaction. Similar fluctuations, Zeki discovered, occurred in the caudate nucleus, found near the center of the brain. The caudate nucleus also activates in response to passionate love; it's the place that integrates more complex thoughts and emotions from different brain regions with the primal, dopamine-fueled rush of desire. The neural maps of our reactions to beauty and to love, then, literally overlap.

The common ground in the processes of love, rejection, and creativity suggests it isn't a very far leap, physiologically speaking, from the pursuit of love to the pursuit of art, particularly for the unrequited lover, who is left empty-handed and unoccupied as the reward of reciprocated love escapes her. One recent study shows that for people who have a high need to feel unique (a common characteristic of artists and innovators), social rejection causes them to score higher on tests of creativity. The outsider identity, which rejection reinforces, nurtures their ability to innovate.

Famed dancer Isadora Duncan insisted that love and art were inextricable, and that she spent her life always "madly in love." As a young dancer living in France, she suffered a double whammy of romantic rejection. She arranged a dinner with champagne and roses for a man she adored, only to watch him rush off in a panic from the romantic scene. She turned in consolation to another suitor, who thrilled her by checking them in to a hotel room under the assumed names of a married couple. Finally, she thought in ecstasy, she would know what love was. But the man backed away, evidently fearful about taking her virginity, and sent her home in a cab. "This last shock," she wrote in her 1927 autobiography *My Life*, "had a decided effect on my emotional nature, turning all its force toward my Art which gave me the joys which Love withheld."

Her connection to dance became more profound. She would stand for hours with her hands folded between her breasts, covering what she came to believe was "the central spring of all movement" in the body. She would develop her highly influential school of dance based on this idea. It was a marked departure from the predominant theory that movement had to stem from the base of the spine—a concept that Duncan said yielded "a mechanical movement not worthy of the soul." The image of Duncan standing in such profound focus and discovery says much about the potential for creativity to arise out of unrequited love. Even if artistic perfection can be as elusive as perfect love, the cycle of reward seeking, dissatisfaction, and satisfaction in making art depends on what the unwanted woman can accomplish herself—not how the beloved responds to her.

THE STORIES OF great artists, I realize, set the bar high. I know from my own experience that the shift from one reward system to another is no magic bullet. There's no recipe for turning the energy of longing into something productive, only examples showing us that it's possible. The euphoric beginning of my obsession, when winning B.'s love seemed possible, did inspire me to write. But after a few months, I was too distracted to work. It was not until after my obsession ended that I could sit down at a desk again. Even then I had to be hours away from him, at an artists' colony in another state where my sole obligation was to write. I wasn't writing for him, and I wasn't writing particularly well. But I was glad to have some focus back.

What my unrequited love inspired, in the end, was not an accomplishment but a change within myself. As I recovered, I made a resolution. "You can't want anyone who isn't good to you," I decided, with the corollary that I had to be able to be good to that person in turn. It was an embarrassingly simple formula, one that I hope my abundantly confident daughter will follow instinctually. If I'd had that rule with B., nothing would have gone past the first indication that he was too confused about his girlfriend to treat me well. I don't know if I would have stopped loving him or prevented myself from becoming obsessed. But I would have kept my respect and sense of self-control. I would have had much less to regret.

With this much needed resolution, my life took a turn that, in retrospect, feels miraculous. Just weeks after B. told me we could never speak again, I met the man who would become my husband. I was very lucky, scoring my life partner on the rebound. I often wonder how I would have fared if I hadn't met Bill. Yet as we slowly built our relationship, my new understanding of myself, and what love should entail, made a difference. I had a standard to go by. I did not want to be the woman who chased too hard again. I needed to make what I had gone through worth something, at least to myself. Later, as I started to deepen my investigation of unrequited love, I met other women who felt that the force of romantic obsession pushed them to change for the better and see their lives anew. The disruptiveness of their unrequited love was in retrospect essential. Their obsession pushed them to where they needed to be.

CAREENA IS A woman who commands notice. She is tall and curvy and always has on the highest heels in the room, giving her an Amazonian presence. She works in public relations and has a digital

Rolodex gilded with celebrities she can convince to do her bidding, often for charity causes; they find her brazenness and Sarah Silverman sense of humor irresistible.

When her son was young, life was a lot quieter. She was restless in her "cushy stay-at-home-mom life." She spent a lot of time shopping and working out at the gym. Her husband of fifteen years had a high-powered advertising job and came home each night preoccupied with work. He wasn't paying much attention to her, and she pointedly told him so. He made an effort—flowers here, compliments there—but he also said he didn't have much time for her. He was too busy making the money she was spending, he explained.

"I'm a pretty tough cookie, and that wasn't going to cut it," she said. "Looking back on it, I probably should have said, 'We should go to couples therapy or look at this with a mediator.' But I didn't do that. Instead, what I did was look across my gym one day and see this very attractive, interesting woman."

"Who is that?" she asked her trainer.

"That," he said, "is trouble."

Careena had never been attracted to women before. "No fooling around, no crushes, no masturbation fantasies where women creep into it. I liked men and sex with men." But there was Sharon, a graduate student ten years younger than she was. Careena walked up, introduced herself, and said, "I have to tell you, I find you captivating. Would you like to have lunch?" She gave Sharon her number and waited with mad impatience the two days it took for her to call. When they met for lunch, one of the first things Careena said was "I'm just going to tell you right away, I'm wildly attracted to you. I don't know why. I know nothing about you. I want to know why I'm attracted to you. I want you to tell me more about yourself."

During Careena's six-month obsession, she and Sharon spent days together while Careena's son was at school. Careena often hired afternoon babysitters so they could be with each other longer. They emailed and texted constantly whenever they were apart. They got matching tattoos. Careena wanted badly to sleep with Sharon. They were affectionate and spent a weekend alone together, sharing the same bed. But Sharon refused to have sex with her. "She was very clear about that," Careena said. "She said, 'There's no way I'm getting involved with a married mother of a child. I'm not going to be your little gay experiment.'"

Careena didn't hide what she was doing from her husband, and he didn't ask her to stop seeing Sharon. "Maybe why she's so important to you is something you need to think about," he said. "I won't stand in your way, but I don't really like the person you're becoming around this." He knew Careena was losing interest in him and pursuing love with someone else. "The intensity was unlike anything that I have ever experienced in my entire life, ever, ever," she said. "I've seen pictures of myself from that time. I'm sparkling. I'm wearing pajamas sitting around someone else's house, and I'm absolutely glowing in the dark."

Careena's frustrated desire eventually became unbearable. As she drove Sharon home after an afternoon they'd spent together, they fought. She told Sharon she didn't want to spend time with her anymore. "I said, 'I can't take it. This is literally killing me. I am torn into a million pieces.'" After Careena dropped Sharon off, Careena went to dinner with a group of mom friends, several of whom knew what she was going through. She was so distraught that she couldn't sit still. She announced, "Either I'm going to stay here and make this all about me or I'm going to leave." They looked at her, not knowing what to say. She went home sobbing and threw herself down on her bed. Her husband came into their bedroom to ask what was wrong. "I hate my life," she said. "Can I help you?" he asked. She said no.

She knew her marriage had to end—and so did her obsession with Sharon. Careena was beginning to realize they wouldn't last as a couple. But the impact of the relationship was profound. She and her husband got divorced not long after, and she moved upstate. Her next serious relationship was with a woman. They've been together eight years, and they recently got married.

Careena resists the simplicity of calling her obsession with Sharon a "coming out story." As Careena describes it, the intensity of her feelings made far more of an impact than the fact that Sharon was female. Yet the drama of Careena's obsessive, impossible love made me think of mid-twentieth-century lesbian pulp fiction. Romantic obsession lured women into same sex affairs, typically with punishing consequences: protagonists driven by unrequited love to suicide, insanity, or depression. When Patricia Highsmith gave the infatuated heroine of her 1952 novel, *The Price of Salt*, a hopeful ending with her female beloved, she offered an alternative vision of the purpose of romantic obsession: that it could lead you to a braver and more truthful existence, even in the face of oppressive social convention.

Careena's unrequited love took place in a far less homophobic time, yet it had a similar force. It pushed her out of a life that no longer felt genuine to her. Her obsession brought out a self-centeredness that drove her to distance herself from what made her unhappy—her marriage and her stay-at-home-mom existence—and court a woman who made her feel alive. Careena's life changed in other ways, too. She had to go back to work after the divorce, and she began to build a career out of the volunteering she'd done during her marriage. "Buying thousand-dollar handbags could never make me as happy as I am now," she said. "My life is harder now, but the clarity and richness are unparalleled." Sharon, The Lover Who Never Was, is still a friend. Careena told me she could telephone Sharon out of the blue and discover they're both playing the same track on the same CD. Sharon was also "the tool that ended my marriage," Careena said. "And I certainly couldn't have reached for a more rocket-red glare tool than that."

ELEANOR, A FIFTY-SIX-YEAR-OLD business consultant in Connecticut, arrived at the emotional wake-up call of unrequited love from a very different place. She had a long and satisfying marriage, enviably infused with a spirit of adventure. After her husband retired and she was laid off unexpectedly from her job, they sold their house in Connecticut and went on a cross-country bicycle trip, starting in Key West and ending in St. Stephen, Canada. Not long after they returned home, he was diagnosed with pancreatic cancer. She spent the next two years helping him fight the disease. "Then I had to give him space to die," she said. "I had to not be angry at him that I would be a widow. It was a huge, difficult journey to take."

After he passed away, she resolved to never let herself love so deeply again. She couldn't stand the thought of being that vulnerable with someone else. She went back to work full-time. She was fifty-four and raising her two grandchildren. "I didn't think I'd have another relationship in my life," she said.

One of her coworkers was a thirty-one-year-old man from India. They were assigned to manage a long-term project. After a year, she realized that she was intensely attracted to him. Her feelings reminded her of the last time she was in unrequited love. She was seventeen and her obsession became self-destructive. "It was like, 'If you won't look at me, just stab me,'" she said. "I thought I was going to drive off a fucking cliff." She became so distraught that she nearly killed herself with a drug overdose. Almost forty years later, as her feelings grew for her colleague, she tried to stifle them. "Here

I am, a year out of being widowed. This just can't be. I don't want to have a crush on this guy. This is not an emotional state I want to be in. But that didn't matter. It became an obsession really quickly."

She knew there was little chance that they could be together. She was white and older than he was, a double taboo in Indian culture. An affair might jeopardize their jobs. Their work relationship, meanwhile, thrived. They had a similar management style: aggressive, fast-paced, not always strict about the rules. She relished his soft-spoken manner and his youthful energy. She was gratified by how comfortable he seemed with her assertiveness.

She realized that instead of feeling devastated over the impossibility of her love, she was enjoying it. Her obsession began to feel like a pleasurable game. "Around him, I'd puff up and slow down my talking," she said. "I would be calmer. I wanted to take it slow, I wanted to be completely present to the sexual energy. At this point in my life, I thought, 'I'm going to wallow in this.'"

Sometimes she felt distraught over her crush, but she found she didn't have much time to wallow in self-pity. Her grandchildren kept her busy when she wasn't at work. When she did have time alone, she fought down the impulse to jump in her car and find him. She knew where he lived and where he hung out with his friends. But she didn't want to act like she had at seventeen. She would let herself occasionally flirt with him on work outings, but that was all.

One afternoon as they were preparing for a presentation, he told Eleanor that he was getting a promotion that would take him back to India. She had known this day would come, but she was devastated. She waited two days, then told him they needed to talk. They sat down in a conference room. "This isn't about how you feel or your response," she said. "This is about what I need to say. I will regret it if I don't say it."

She carefully told him how she felt. He took a deep breath and told her he didn't want to hurt her. She assured him that she needed nothing from him. "You don't have responsibility for my heartbreak," she said. "This is what my heart has done. I didn't think I could feel this way again after losing my husband, and it's really good for me to know I can go to this place with someone." She knew she couldn't think about love as something she could avoid for the rest of her life. She was capable of getting close to someone else. She wanted another relationship, even if it wasn't with him.

He received her confession calmly. He told her he would never forget her. As she suspected, he had nothing more to give her—no confession of mutual desire, no eleventh-hour fling. A few nights later, they went out to dinner, and their rapport was still there. They parted as friends.

WHAT STRIKES ME about Eleanor is how determined she was not to fall prey to her unrequited love. She couldn't control her feelings, but she could control how she acted in response to them—and let them move her to a new understanding of what her future could bring. "I have thrown myself off the ledge before, and I decided I wasn't going to do it this time," she said. "What I have to hold on to now is much more important to me than if I had actually gone to bed with him."

Eleanor's story shows that the unwanted woman can use what she's going through for a larger purpose. She can know what she wants isn't possible. She can fantasize, knowing that her fantasies will never be real. She can experience love without real expectations—and with a Don Quixote freedom to do what she needs to do with the feeling. Clinical psychologist Jill Weber, the author of *Having Sex, Wanting Intimacy: Why Women Settle for*

One-Sided Relationships, says women may be drawn to unrequited love in times of transition. "They are trying to figure something out," she said. "They're not ready for commitment, but this allows them to feel desire at a distance without risking rejection. It's what the self needs to do." As in the preadolescent and teen years, unrequited love can be a necessary phase for an adult, helping her learn—or relearn—how to love within the relative safety of a one-sided attraction.

The key for Eleanor was adult-size restraint, which seems anathema to passion. She put rules around her obsession and, within those rules, found pleasure and insight. Social psychologist Sharon Brehm has observed a similar phenomenon in religious traditions, which place ecstatic spiritual love "within the context of a disciplined life of devotion." The sixteenth-century nun Teresa of Ávila wrote of mood swings that went from euphoria to despair to blank exhaustion as she experienced love for an unknowable God. She felt mystical moments of union, "like rain falling from the heavens into a river," as well as times of panic when she could not feel as close to God as she wanted. All this took place within a life of strict discipline, untenable to most of us. But there is something important in the combination of order and disorder that characterized Teresa of Ávila's ecstasy—and, in a thoroughly contemporary and a-religious manner, Eleanor's approach to her crush. Eleanor worked with her passion and let it teach her. We don't have to become nuns. We don't have to stifle all feeling. But we may need to learn, as individuals and as a culture, ways to honor passion by confining and using it instead of letting it diminish us.

9

Letting Go

HOW OBSESSION ENDS

◆

B. HAD NOT ANSWERED HIS PHONE IN days. One morning I tried him from my office at school.

"Phillips," he said as soon as he heard my voice, "I'm cutting you off. We can never speak again." He hung up.

I canceled my classes for the rest of the day. I went back to my apartment and got into bed. I felt weak and had a fever. The next morning, I vomited. Immediately after, I felt, if not normal, that I could glimpse normalcy. My temperature went back down. I was no longer possessed. I was shaken and alone. I had failed, but I could move forward.

That twenty-four-hour flu was my exorcism.

The demon was gone. The end of my obsession began with the words "we can never speak again." B. ended all possibility. He had never done that before.

I was ready. At long last, I had to accept the repeated rejections, the girlfriend he couldn't bring himself to leave, the simple fact that after six months of strenuous effort, we still weren't together. Dorothy Tennov would have called what I went through *starvation*—the lack of consistent attention and caring from B., on top of all the accumulated evidence that a relationship wasn't going to happen. After that final phone call, I no longer had anything to feed my hopes. A couple of weeks later, I left Pittsburgh for a while. The trip, planned before my obsession began, was fortuitous. I needed to wake up with a couple hundred miles between us instead of a few blocks.

Finding distance, in real miles or metaphorical ones, can be crucial to ending romantic obsession. Maria, the woman obsessed with a man who worked at a sporting-goods store a few miles south of her home, stopped driving by the store. Even the sight of it, she knew, would retrigger her attraction, making her miserable. She did all her errands in the other direction.

A CONCLUSIVE REJECTION that ends all contact, as heartless as it might seem, is a blessing for the unwanted woman whose obsession has become compulsive, demoralizing, or destructive. Ambivalence and mixed messages are her curse. So are the intermittent positive rewards of sex, affection, friendship, and other kinds of attention. When people confide in me that they are being aggressively pursued, I tell them the story of my final phone call with B. I urge them to be as unequivocal as he finally was. When unrequited love gets out of hand, the moral dilemma of the beloved boils down to this: Rejection is mercy.

There are limits to this idea. Plenty of aspiring lovers persist beyond an unequivocal no. And plenty of beloveds won't or can't be so clear. The unwanted woman who wants to stop being consumed by unrequited love may need another way out, a way that isn't dependent on what the beloved does.

How, then, does romantic obsession end?

Just as there are many ways to be in obsessive love, there are many ways to get out of it, though common themes and larger lessons do emerge. Most of the women in this book (including me) didn't follow any one particular strategy or program. Some found solace in support groups. Some got professional help, an option people whose obsession is limiting their ability to function or spurring them to destructive behavior should seek. Rest assured, with rare exceptions, unrequited love does end.

ONE OF THE legs that unrequited love stands on is the importance of the beloved—all the goals and dreams you've imbued him with. The goals and dreams don't have to end, but their association with the beloved does. Renowned physician Ibn Sina realized this back in the tenth century, when he prescribed refuting the lovesick patient's idealized notions as "nothing but a delusion" and pointing out the beloved's character flaws. Take the magic away. Unlink the goals, dissolve the crystals. He also advised strenuous distractions: hunting, intellectual debates, and other physically and mentally challenging activities.

Ibn Sina's remedy, as psychologist Frank Tallis points out, is echoed today in a number of therapeutic approaches rooted in cognitive behavioral therapy (CBT). CBT helps people identify and change the beliefs that direct self-destructive and self-defeating thoughts and actions. If you believe the beloved is the only man on earth who can give you the love you need and you *must* be with him, you'll continue to behave accordingly. CBT prompts the patient to challenge the strength of the belief: How, for example, could your beloved be the only man who can give you the love you need if he doesn't text you back? How could he be fulfilling his long-ago promise to spend his life with you if he won't even agree to let you see him?

Several CBT-based approaches emphasize disrupting the unsatisfying cycle of the reward-seeking behaviors of obsessive love. You may look for solace in photos of your beloved, but the relief is only momentary. The more you give in to the impulse, the more accustomed your brain becomes to this quick yet weak dose of reassurance. It becomes a habit that feels crucial to your very survival. Not long after you stop gazing at the picture, or even while you're still looking at it, the craving to reconnect builds again. Cognitive behavioral therapy essentially guides patients to recognize the craving as misguided urgings of their brain—not the call of a truly essential need—and then directs their attention to an activity or thought that's more beneficial. This approach taps in to the brain's neuroplasticity, the capacity to take on new roles and functions in response to changes in the brain's environment. CBT, in short, can literally transform the way the brain works. A small study of patients with obsessive-compulsive disorder found that after ten weeks of CBT, two thirds of the patients suffered fewer OCD symptoms—and their brain chemistry shifted accordingly. When OCD symptoms are intense, more glucose is metabolized in the area of the brain that signals when something has gone wrong with an expected reward. After the treatment, glucose metabolism in that area decreased, along with the symptoms.

Los Angeles–based clinical psychologist Jennifer Taitz uses a CBT-based technique to help her clients gain more control over their thoughts and their behavior. "People think that if they have a desire, they need to act on it. They think it's cathartic to send an email or talk about the person. But that's a myth," she said. "If you change your behavior, you can change the way you feel. If you don't talk about him, your feelings may pass faster, and you'll surely live better." She teaches a tool called "Opposite to Emotion Action." Instead of giving in to the urge to satisfy your desire to connect, you "gently avoid" it and do the opposite: Put away the pictures, delete the person's number, and refrain from talking about him.

Key to Taitz's process is having her patients focus on values. She asks them to assess what they want out of life. Her therapeutic approach helps them move toward a renewed commitment to their personal values. "Values motivate people," she said. "If someone values integrity and can really look at that, that can help more than anything else." Assessing values helps them see that their struggle is for something bigger and better in their life—*not* the particular person they've been obsessing over. "If people realize that they care about taking care of themselves and having compassion for themselves, they'll see that they are not going to get those things by seeing someone whose love is not reciprocal."

Taitz's approach struck me as a concrete way to dismantle goal linking by guiding the patient to see how her higher-order goals have little to do with the lower-order goal of a relationship with the beloved. Taitz emphasized that moving beyond the fixation on the beloved can be a "really tortuous and really brutal" process, but keeping your values in mind can help. "It's almost like a firefighter goes into a building and is willing to endure the flames to rescue a baby," she said.

For several of the women I interviewed, the beliefs they once had about their beloved dissolved in an abrupt epiphany, as if the curtain had been drawn back on their Wizard of Oz and he was revealed to be nothing more than human—and not the right human for them to love. Some of these turning points seem, like my fever, sent from some divine place, as if Aphrodite and Athena agreed that it was time for the madness to cease. One woman's obsession ended in the Oakland firestorm of 1991. Her home burned down, and all her possessions were destroyed. She and her husband had to focus on basic needs: consoling their son, finding a place to live, buying underwear and toothpaste. Her unrequited love, for months the guiding force for everything she did, seemed extraneous. The fire "was a cleansing," she said. "You lose your history, and you're down to just your physical being. You don't have your stuff anymore. The facade of the drama, the passion, was part of that stuff. You get down to your core life."

Other women undergo a long, gradual process before their moment of realization. Amalia, a fifty-four-year-old inn owner, spent her early twenties obsessed with Rick, a close friend she met while working at a restaurant. He had a drawn, bony face ("like Daniel Day-Lewis in *The Unbearable Lightness of Being*") and a tortured spirit, a seductive combination for her and, she suspected, many others. They were roommates and occasional lovers, but he always pulled away from her when he sensed she wanted too much. She believed she represented stability and unconditional love as he immersed himself in the creative ferment of film school in New York City. She was more grounded than he was; plus, she had a dog they both adored.

When living together became too fraught, they decided he should move out. She nursed hopes that once he left, their relationship would grow stronger. Then she discovered she was pregnant. He urged her to get an abortion. After a lot of soul-searching, she reluctantly went ahead with terminating the pregnancy. He stayed with her throughout the procedure and cared for her afterward. "Then he began to extricate himself from me, even from our friendship," she said. A few months after she lost touch with him, she spotted him as she was heading into a movie theater in midtown Manhattan to see *The Last Métro*. The sight of him across the avenue, laughing and happy with a friend, made her feel so ill that she couldn't make it through the movie. She got into a cab and threw up all over the seat.

She didn't see Rick again for about two years. She got married and had a baby son. One morning, as she was strolling her baby on Manhattan's Upper East Side, she spotted Rick riding on his bicycle and waved. As he approached, she watched him, fascinated. She knew she didn't love him anymore. But not long before that morning, her husband had mentioned his name—they both worked in the film industry—and she'd felt her heart twinge with the memory of what he had meant to her.

She greeted him warmly. "This is my son," she said. "You're not going to believe what I named him!"

"Rick?"

"What?" she gasped, startled.

In that moment, she told me, she saw him for who he really was in a way she never could when she was in love with him. "There was something so heinous and narcissistic in his belief that I would actually *name my child after him*! I saw how ludicrous he was—he thought I still had that much unresolved feeling for him. It blew me away. I already felt I had moved on, and I was grateful for where I was at in life. But if I had any feeling left for him, it vaporized in that moment. It was the ultimate closure."

She graciously corrected him. "No, Rick. I named him Monte." It was the name of the dog she had when they lived together.

Like Amalia, Rina, the opera singer, took years to get over her love for her college conductor. She saw him from time to time in the music world, and their encounters were often disappointing, sometimes devastatingly so. At graduate school, she was thrilled to learn he would be visiting for a professional meeting. When she spotted his bobbing walk in the distance, she called out to him. She was certain he heard her, but he ignored her and walked in the opposite direction. At his conducting debut with a major symphony orchestra, she went backstage to congratulate him. She found herself in a throng of many "adoring female acolytes" who, she suspected, felt for him as she had. "To see them all assembled made me feel embarrassed and pathetic," she said.

Then her own career began to take off. She was asked to perform an orchestral song cycle by Leonard Bernstein at a prestigious music festival. The lyrics, a poem by Conrad Aiken, were all about lost love: "Music I heard with you was more than music / And bread I broke with you was more than bread / Now that I am without you, all is desolate / All that was once so beautiful is dead." While she rehearsed the piece, she sometimes choked up, thinking of the conductor. In performance, she was flawless. The song cycle was met with a thunderous ovation. Afterward, to her utter surprise, her beloved conductor walked through the backstage door and embraced her. "It was a triumph on my own terms," she said. "I now had the bravery to sing without emotions overcoming me. It was a good apotheosis and really allowed me to let go." She didn't need him in order to become the performer she wanted to be, and the idea of him no longer held the same power.

THERE ARE WAYS to catalyze the moment of awakening that ends romantic obsession. Emma, a documentary filmmaker, began practicing Buddhism in her early thirties. Her teacher, a monk named Peter, suggested she move into the Zen monastery where he worked. The idea of a semi-monastic existence appealed to her. She had been bedridden for several weeks with chicken pox, followed by a bout of mononucleosis. The isolation of being sick for so long had left her with the feeling that something was "profoundly missing" from her life. Though her career was showing strong signs of promise, her parents didn't really understand what she was doing. She was burdened with the feeling that she wasn't meeting their expectations. Deepening her practice at the monastery offered solace. "You bring your hands together, and it's like a wake-up bell," she said. "There's a way you become very, very close to people when you sit in silence for hours on end."

The monastery had a strict rule for newcomers: no relationships for the first six months. "They've seen that when people first move in, they are very sensitive and more vulnerable than they normally are," Emma said.

The restriction didn't stop her from becoming obsessed with Jack, a senior monk. When she sat down to meditate at five each morning, all she could think about was having sex with him. Buddhist monks don't have to be celibate, and she knew Jack wanted her, too. She took her dilemma to her teacher. "I know there's this six-month rule, but I just want to hop into the sack with this guy," she confessed. "I can't stop thinking about him. We're made for each other."

Her teacher, Peter, told her a story. In his twenties, he traveled to Asia to escape the violence in his native Ireland and seek enlightenment. He moved into a monastery in a remote forest in Thailand, but all he could think about was raunchy sex. Pornographic scenes invaded his meditation. He went to his teacher for help. The teacher sent him to live in a brothel for a year. His explanation was that he needed to "study desire."

Emma was shocked. "Did you have sex?" she asked. Peter said that at first he did. But then the prostitutes started seeking his friendship. They shared with him the pain in their lives. "I became their brother," he said. "I couldn't objectify them, and I couldn't see them in this raunchy and sexy way." He stopped sleeping with the prostitutes, and his lust faded.

Then Peter gave Emma his advice. "If you want to have sex with Jack, have sex with Jack. But wait two weeks. Try studying your desire."

She followed his advice. The more she held back, the more Jack pursued her. There were no locks on the bedroom doors, and he would wait naked in her room for her. But she didn't give in. She began to see him more clearly. "It was like being zoomed in on a close-up shot, and then the lens slowly opens up to a medium shot, and I saw all these layers of him I couldn't see before because we weren't sleeping together," she said. "This nuance gets crushed once you go fuck someone. You just want to merge."

Her longing for him, she realized, was about an ideal, not a reality. "The more I felt I had to be with him, the more I was not really seeing him," she said. "I was focused on how I was finally going to feel once I was with him. I was finally going to be really myself. I was finally going to land in the world."

Once she studied her desire, she realized how unrealistic that line of thinking was—and how little she felt for him. "It's always simpler, the way you fantasize about it," she said. "You don't fantasize about the messiness of intimacy. It never includes the stuff that really gets on your nerves. It filters all that out. I took what was attractive about him and purified it and imagined that being with him was somehow going to make me feel whole."

What Emma learned—to sit with her feelings instead of acting on them—is part of the strategy behind dialectical behavior therapy (DBT). Developed by psychologist Marsha Linehan to treat chronically suicidal women, DBT emphasizes both self-acceptance and the need to change destructive behaviors. DBT programs combine individual therapy sessions with phone coaching and skills groups to help clients learn how to manage anger, depression, impulsivity, stress, relationships, and other challenges. Barry Rosenfeld, a psychology professor at Fordham University, created a stalking treatment program that uses DBT. Participants, all criminal offenders who are court-ordered to participate in treatment, are taught to use mindfulness techniques to observe their urges to contact the target of their harassment without acting on them. "A lot of offenders are just not accustomed to thinking before they act," Rosenfeld said. "A lot of people are very impulsive. Something happens, and then they do something to react. We are trying to break that chain and get people to tolerate feeling bad and not go right into action to stop feeling bad." None of the people who completed Rosenfeld's pilot program were arrested again for a stalking offense, while nearly half of all convicted stalkers overall reoffend.

This idea—of learning how to sit with your feelings—is useful in controlling less extreme forms of pursuit. It's at the heart of the approach developed by Rhonda Findling, who counsels women all over the world about how to stop the obsessive urge to connect and get over romantic obsession. She recently developed a "Don't Text That Man" app that helps you keep track of the last time you contacted your beloved. The app delivers encouraging bits of advice: "Isn't it better to be the girl who got away rather than the clingy desperate girl?" The approach may be a bit techno-cheesy, but I view Findling as a valuable figure in the self-help world. She doesn't shame women about not being feminine enough, and she doesn't tell them not to initiate relationships. Rather, she urges them to stop compulsive pursuit and regain self-control. Her core message is an important one: You have to learn to tolerate your distress. Otherwise, you'll become masochistic, offering yourself up again and again to the pain of rejection. "What you have to do is go against the grain," Findling said. "You're thinking, 'He has to see how much I love and desire him!' Containing your feelings and waiting doesn't feel natural. It goes against the instinct."

For self-control to work, she said, women need to "suffer out" their pain instead of contacting the beloved in an effort to get rid of it. When your beloved doesn't respond to you, that in itself is a real loss. It doesn't matter how long the relationship lasted or whether there was ever a "real" relationship. You need to allow yourself to mourn, just as anyone who has lost someone important needs to mourn. She tells women to expect to go through stages much like Elisabeth Kübler-Ross described in her famous 1969 book, *On Death and Dying*: denial, anger, bargaining, depression, and acceptance. They will need similar forms of support: friends they can confide in, creative outlets, structured time, physical exercise. If you need to express your feelings, Findling suggests you write the beloved a letter. Just don't send it.

Some women, however, are released from obsession precisely *because* they had a chance to communicate what they felt to their beloved. Carolyn, the young woman who was obsessed with her art school classmate, found solace after she gave him a diary of her feelings. Sonya, the design researcher, struggled with her feelings after months of mixed signals and disappointments. She had never overtly pursued her beloved. She had never told him how much she cared about him and how much he had angered her. Once she carefully confessed to him, the last traces of her obsession went away. The difference between the unwanted woman who needs to stop connecting and the one who needs to connect lies in her degree of self-control and her level of expectation. Carolyn and Sonya reached out after they had stopped hoping for love or, for that matter, any particular response. They needed to unburden themselves of what they were feeling, and they did so with dignity. Los Angeles clinical psychologist Jennifer Taitz cautioned that though this approach can be helpful for some people, it's risky. "It can backfire and trigger a mini-relapse," she said. "The thing that I say to people is: 'Do you want to be right or live a good life?'"

Over a year after my obsession with B. subsided, I went back to Pittsburgh for a visit. My friends and I drove around the city on a Saturday night, looking for a place to have coffee. Every favorite haunt was too crowded or closed. We decided to go to the Squirrel Hill café in my old neighborhood, where B. and I had spent a lot of time. I had wanted to avoid it, but the longer we searched for a suitable place, the more inevitable it seemed. Indeed, when we walked in, B. was sitting at a table near the door with a group of my favorite students from my last year teaching in Pittsburgh. After I caught up with my students, I invited B. to sit with me at another table. I told him I was working in radio again and living in Woodstock with Bill. B. said he had been wondering where I went. He knew I left town because he stopped hearing me on the radio on Saturday mornings. It was nice to be the one who disappeared mysteriously, leaving him guessing, I thought.

We talked about what had gone on between us. He said he was still trying to figure out why he acted the way he did. I said I regretted what I had become. It wasn't like me to be a crazed stalker, I said wryly.

We smiled at each other. I experienced a faint reprise of the old attraction, though I knew I wouldn't act on it. I felt self-possessed again, the way I did when we were classmates, when I was mildly attracted to him but hadn't given him any power over me. I'd made my comeback from the wreck I'd been. I was building a good, sane life without him. Facing him from that vantage point gave me some of the thrill of what I might call revenge, but none of the consequences.

And so I return to the question that launched this book: Why did I *ever* give him all that power? Why did I get so obsessed? My outsize reaction to being unwanted didn't, as far as I can determine, stem from an early psychological wound or malfunction of attachment. What sent me into the psychological and neurochemical maelstrom I've detailed in these pages was nothing that exceptional: I was lost. I'd suffered a breakup of a serious relationship—a major predictor of unwanted pursuit. I'd had several bouts of anxiety and depression since my teens and was desperate to avoid another one. My teaching job was temporary, my radio job part-time, and my writing was in a post–graduate school no-man's-land. I didn't know what I was going to do with my career. Several of my closest friends were leaving Pittsburgh, getting married, having children, or moving in with someone. Both my siblings had growing families. I had lived in five different states during my twenties, moving with a kind of erratic determination between going to school and radio jobs. I was weary of starting over yet again and of being on my own.

My life illustrated the downside of what social scientists now call extended adolescence. Delaying family and a settled profession—the markers of "adult life"—has its freedoms and pleasures. But such a prolonged period of uncertainty (exacerbated by an economy that increasingly feeds off of part-time, contract, and internship labor, none of which requite workers' longings for commitment) can also engender despair. I felt lonely and ashamed. Despite my heartfelt efforts in work and love, nothing I did seemed to amount to much. None of these challenges—all common and very human—were insurmountable. But their combined force made me vulnerable when I drew close to B., a man who at first saw me as I so badly wanted to see myself: smart, desirable, strong.

MEETING MY HUSBAND SO soon after B. cut me off gave me what I was chasing so hard: the self-esteem that comes from being wanted by a good man, followed by love, marriage, and a family. I don't want this to sound smug or easy. Early in my relationship with Bill, I returned to therapy to help myself become more emotionally self-reliant. However supportive Bill was, I was dealing with many of the same life challenges I had before I met him, and I had to realize that he wasn't responsible for fixing them all. For our love to endure, I had to shake off the illusion that his attention was going to take care of my well-being as I sorted my life out. As a girl who came of age in the era of *The Cinderella Complex*, I had never bought into the idea that a man should provide for all my material needs. Yet until this turning point in my life, the myth persisted that a partner would provide completely for my emotional security.

My relationship with Bill meant I skipped a very difficult stage endured by many people coping with unrequited love: walking into the future without a partner. But that doesn't have to mean walking into the future without love. The role of good love in easing a failed obsession isn't limited to replacement romances. Caroline Hostetler, a behavioral neuroscientist at Oregon Health & Science University, studies the impact of social attachment on addictive disorders. She takes issue with researchers who maintain that because the neural processes of love, social attachment, and addiction have so much in common, the same pharmacological treatments for addiction might apply to people suffering from the loss of love. This line of thinking, she says, misses a crucial point: Social attachments are necessary to our welfare, whereas drugs and alcohol are not. The fact that both social attachments and substance abuse trigger reward systems suggests that quality relationships of all sorts can neurologically "compete" with substance addiction. "Maybe social relationships can be the more powerful addiction," she says.

The obsessed lover is caught in a bind when her quest for attachment to the beloved becomes unhealthy and compulsive. Seeking other human connections—supportive family and friends, therapy groups, community—can help give her addiction to him some healthy neurochemical competition.

MELISSA, A FIFTY-EIGHT-YEAR-OLD office manager, was in an obsessive, on-again, off-again affair with Gordon for three years. Two months after they got together, she found out that he was seeing another woman. He described it as a temporary relationship. Then Melissa found out he had been with her for two years and owned a house with her. The news tore Melissa up. She spent months crying and writing letters to him that she never sent. The only comfort she could find seemed to be with him. Their affair resumed. "I should have run, but I didn't," she said.

At first they spent every weekend together, fishing on his boat. Melissa loved the peacefulness of being out on the water with him and having him all to herself. When his girlfriend found out what was going on, Gordon told Melissa that she didn't mind. Melissa started to, though. "He could have her and me, too, and I felt cheated," she said. "I began to lose my confidence and self-respect." Even though she tried to stop seeing Gordon, she let the affair drag out for four years. "I just turned into a dead person. I wasn't doing anything but living for him and going to work so I could survive."

Then she felt the pull of a different kind of attachment. Her brother, who lived in Florida and suffered from schizophrenia and advancing dementia, was dying. She decided to leave Tennessee to be with him and her sister, who lived nearby and would help with his care. "That became my priority," she said. "I knew my relationship wasn't giving anything to me anymore, and I knew if I didn't leave, I'd be stuck indefinitely in the twilight zone, doing the same thing over and over again. I didn't want to leave, but I just felt I had to. I couldn't go on."

She sold her house and left the state. "I knew I could do this thing—move away and leave him and care for my brother," she said. "I could be the winner a little bit." For the next two years, she was swept up in her brother's needs. He required constant care. "He was always after attention from doctors, nurses, me," she said. "I could never stop to rest or relax." Although it was exhausting, it broke her tie to Gordon. "I focused on my brother rather than myself and how sad and lonely I felt." The move, which brought her closer to other family members, made her feel more confident and stable. All she had to do was look at her brother, who needed her so much. Everything she'd been through with Gordon felt "a little silly" in comparison. This renewed human connection could sustain her as she finally gained distance from Gordon.

Psychologists call heartbreak "social pain." Rejection hurts so much because we've lost a social connection. Social pain is an adaptation. Our ancestors needed other people to protect themselves from wild animals, hostile tribes, and the elements. To be excluded from a community was a life-threatening proposition, so the strife of being rejected had to push people to respond as they would to a physical injury: They had to do something to repair it. Social pain and physical pain involve similar areas of the brain and cause similar reactions—weeping, screaming, seeking help. The caring presence of other people helps alleviate hurt feelings *and* physical pain; several studies show that higher levels of social support are associated with lower levels of pain in labor, after surgery, and in people suffering from chronic pain and heart disease. Melissa could, in today's terms, "take care of herself"—she'd been on her own for years. But what helped ease the blow of rejection was reconnecting with her siblings. They needed her, and she needed them.

Loved ones and other forms of social attachment are crucial, helping us fend off all manner of challenges to our ability to thrive. In a society where more people live alone than ever before, it's easy to forget that closeness to others isn't a luxury, something to seek out when we don't have anything else to do. It's tempting to live out too much of our social lives online, at the expense of real-life human contact. If we isolate ourselves, we risk being all the more vulnerable when someone walks into our lives and triggers all that unsatisfied need.

Yet there is no question that social attachments to family and friends are very different from romantic love. Even the best strategies for ending romantic obsession can feel very much like paces to put yourself through, emotional homework: necessary but not nearly as exciting as what we left behind. They're meant to help us stop suffering. But they can seem to require us to stop living so large, so unrealistically. We must become *sensible.* The pull of unrequited love can stem from a longing for transcendence, a need to experience great, impractical feeling. So for some of us, moving beyond obsession may entail finding something or someone with a similar ineffable power.

Lina, an Italian-language specialist and forty-six-year-old single mother, expressed this idea perfectly in a bit of woodsy folklore: "They say the antidote grows right next to the poison."

Lina is exactly the kind of person I'm talking about. She does need to live large, whether by investigating the intricacies of Italian etymology or immersing herself in a new and enchanting friendship. She has a sharp, analytical mind and a mystical emotional sensibility guided by moments of synchronicity. Her daughter was conceived with a man she had spent a passionate night with in a lightning storm. He lived in Greece and saw his daughter only sporadically. Lina cherished her daughter, but raising her alone was difficult. She had little money and little help; her parents had died when she was in her twenties.

She met Bartolo through a mutual friend when he was visiting from Italy. They connected immediately over their mutual interest in languages, "geeking out" over etymology and the connections among Italian, Greek, Latin, and Sanskrit. They soon discovered that they were born on the same day, three hours apart, which Lina took as a sign that "there was something bigger at work"— they were meant to be together. She nursed that feeling for two years, despite the fact that Bartolo disappointed her again and again. When she and her daughter visited him in Italy, he became jealous of the four-year-old girl and kicked them out of his home. On a trip to Romania, he abandoned her after a disagreement and sent a text to let her know where he'd moved her luggage. They got together again in Mexico. Finally, Lina said, everything felt "perfect, a honeymoon." Then his attention wandered to a Venetian woman they'd met in a restaurant. At the end of the trip, when he put Lina on a bus to the airport instead of driving her there, she knew he planned to seek the woman out. Lina's love for Bartolo, she realized, left her in a "constant state of longing." It had to come to an end.

Lina sat down in a daze in the airport lounge. She wondered what was going to become of her life. She was depleted emotionally and financially. Then a "beautiful blue-eyed" man sat down three chairs away from her. "That's when everything changed," she said.

She started talking to the man, whose name was Oliver. When they got in line to board the plane, they realized that they were seated next to each other. "What are the chances of that?" she said, and laughed. She made him show her his ticket to prove it. Oliver, an economics researcher, counted the number of seats on the plane and, to her delight, started calculating the odds. They talked all the way home. When she learned that he was twenty years younger than she was, she found it "incomprehensible that there could be such an old soul in a young body."

As she described how quickly her feelings for him developed—an "immediate, unconditional" love—I feared she was telling a story of replacing one unrealistic love with another. But she assured me there was a critical difference: She didn't need anything from Oliver.

They kept in touch. She cut her ties to Bartolo. Meeting Oliver "created a new standard" for her. "I asked myself, would I want the kind of relationship I had with Bartolo for my daughter? That's a simple one. I would not want this for my daughter."

One day she received a text from Oliver's roommate. Oliver had been in a motorcycle accident. He was in a coma and might not live. As soon as she could, Lina drove down to Baltimore from her home in upstate New York.

At the hospital, Oliver's family members, believing he wasn't going to make it, were coming in to say goodbye. "They were speaking about him in the third person, in the past tense, as if he was already gone," she said. "Things like: 'Oliver was so good at the piano, Oliver was this, Oliver was that.' They were living their greatest fear."

When she had a moment alone with Oliver, she touched his ears and stroked his cheekbone. She whispered to him, "I haven't had time to tell you how I feel because I haven't known you long enough, but I have this difficult-to-explain love for you. I want you to understand there are things for you to do here."

Lina left the hospital not knowing what was going to happen. But on her drive home, she got a text from his roommate: "He opened his eyes." A few days later, Oliver was well enough to try to talk his doctors into letting him leave the hospital. She felt her presence had been a part of what saved him.

During his recovery, I asked her, "If he called you tomorrow and said he didn't want to see you again, would you be okay?"

"Yes," she said. "I can feel for him with no boundaries, because I have no expectations."

Indeed, Lina never had a romance with Oliver. In the two years since his recovery, he has visited her several times. He shares a close bond with her daughter, whom he fondly calls his "niece." He helps Lina around her house and property and with her writing. "I'm an older woman he trusts," she said. They've tested the boundaries of their friendship; on one visit they fooled around. But she quickly realized their relationship wasn't meant to be sexual. The very fact that she and Oliver never became a couple and, she feels, probably never could be, has great meaning for her. "Oliver primes me for great love," she said. "To love, I have to take care of my own emotional life, and he helps me do that."

One of the easiest ways to deal with unrequited love is to dismiss it as a delusion, a dream that takes us nowhere. I think this is the easy way out. We don't have to tell ourselves we can't get anything out of the state of being in love unless it becomes a full-blown romance. As Lina's story shows, there are many in-between ways of being in love—her feeling for Oliver is more than a friendship, but it's not a romance, either. For that matter, it's not unrequited love, but it shows us what unrequited love can be at its best: intense, fruitful *feeling*, without expectations.

Lina's daughter is a year younger than Clara. As Lina and I spoke in my living room one morning, the two girls played upstairs, making scary movies on my cell phone. They rushed down to show us what they'd done. On the phone's small screen, Lina and I watched their serious, horrified faces, their hair Sunday-morning-messy, their costumes a whimsical combination of camouflage and scissored-up Halloween garb. They were in that period of girlhood I remember so well, when imaginary play is all-consuming and a good book can take over the world on weekend afternoons. The idea of romantic love was still fairly incomprehensible to them, but it wouldn't stay that way much longer.

I know that secure love and care now will help my daughter weather the storm later, hopefully with the same strong sense of self that she carries into her current friendships. I've also come to believe that our society as a whole could do a better job raising children to have healthy romantic relationships. We have a great deal at stake in learning to love. Good relationships are a major factor in quality of life, mortality rates, and happiness. Yet we leave courtship—the way relationships begin—largely in "the vast realm of cultural mystery," said Brian Spitzberg, a communication professor at San Diego State University and a leading researcher on obsessive romantic pursuit. "We don't teach it in school. It's not seen as an appropriate area of instruction. We allow people to learn it through trial and error, an extremely inefficient way of learning. There are all sorts of ambiguities in the process. We lose track of the bigger picture of what makes better relationships because we're trying to decode all the signals. We're trying to figure out how the other person feels and regulate our own emotions."

A quality relationship ed program won't eliminate unrequited love—and I wouldn't want to eliminate it completely, given the beneficial role played by certain kinds of unrequited love in our lives. But if we can teach kids about sex in high school classrooms, is it so outlandish to propose that we also teach them about the human tendency to get romantically obsessed, what it might mean, and how to handle it with dignity? Can't we teach them about ways to cope with unrequited attraction and obsession—and how, when they're ready, to let it go?

From the time Clara was quite small, I've found opportunities to talk about love and relationships, bringing in what I've discovered in the process of writing this book. When Clara was a kindergartener, she loved *Peanuts*, a comic strip that is all about unrequited love. Charlie Brown once famously bemoaned, "Nothing takes the taste out of peanut butter quite like unrequited love." The strip links its characters in chains of unreturned adoration. Peppermint Patty loves Charlie Brown, Charlie Brown loves the Little Red-Haired Girl. Sally loves Linus, who loves his teacher, Miss Othmar. Lucy loves Schroeder, who wants nothing more than to play Beethoven on his toy piano.

In one of the comic strips, Lucy leans on the piano, asking Schroeder to tell her she's beautiful. When he doesn't, she announces, "If I go out of your life, it will become empty, and all your practicing will be as pursuing the wind." Without lifting his gaze from the piano, he replies, "Try me!"

But Lucy doesn't leave. She kicks the piano, believing the instrument to be her rival, the only thing standing in the way of Schroeder's love. When that doesn't do much, she flings the piano into the "dreaded kite-eating tree," which chomps the instrument to dust.

When Clara burst out laughing, I didn't try to stifle her glee. It's a comic, after all. But I didn't want the menace of the situation to go unnoticed, so I said, "It's really mean, what Lucy did. Schroeder loved his piano." Lucy is a lot more than an unwanted girl who went too far: She's authoritative, smart, and enterprising, with a lemonade-stand-style "psychiatrist help" booth advertising a nickel a session. It's significant that the strip combines these qualities with her inclination to be rude and manipulative, suggesting that female ambition and the capacity for emotional violation go hand in hand. But this was something, I told myself, that I could bring up when Clara was older, if the opportunity arose. In that moment, the idea of "mean," which any five-year-old can understand, would be enough. Clara nodded. "Read some more," she said, eager, as always, to find something else that would make her giggle.

As Clara approaches adolescence, I've shared bits of my own story of obsession, in greatly watered-down form, as a cautionary tale—though she insists she doesn't need it. "I'm not going to get obsessed with a boy like you did, Mommy," she's told me pointedly, more than once. She may indeed be right. If she's not, I hope I can be helpful—though I'm well aware of the tendency of kids to ignore their parents' advice (even if they've authored a book about the subject!) or hide what they're going through. For now, I have to believe that keeping the unrequited love awareness campaign going in a casual and open way just might do some good.

Acknowledgments

MY FIRST THANK-YOU GOES TO MY ED-
itor, Gail Winston, whose keen insights and
suggestions were fundamental throughout.
She pushed me when I need to be pushed, in
all the right ways. I also thank my agent, Henry
Dunow, who recognized the promise of this
project early on and offered abundant sage advice on how to turn it into a book. Dan Jones,
the editor of the "Modern Love" column of *The
New York Times*, helped me see back in 2006
that strong reactions to unrequited love are
common and very human. My editing sessions
with him were great therapy, which he graciously didn't charge me a dime for.

Like many writers, I wrote this book while
juggling a full-time job and family life. I am
grateful to Yaddo, the Virginia Center for
the Creative Arts, the Millay Colony, and

Jentel for concentrated periods of time to focus on my writing. With the volume turned down on the rest of my life, I could nurture this project with patience and clarity. I also thank my employer, SUNY New Paltz, for supporting *Unrequited* through a pre-tenure fellowship leave and a research and creative projects grant. My students at New Paltz kept me connected to the fast-changing world of social media and the trials of young people in the mating game. They cheered me on and eagerly followed my progress, which meant so much to me. I thank student assistants Beth Curran and Lauren Scrudato for their help with transcribing and research.

I received mentoring and encouragement from Melanie Thernstrom, Kenneth Wapner, and Gail Bradney. I cherish the conversations about unrequited love that I had with Emily Bauman, Jaime Karnes, Elizabeth Thompson, Andrew Gebert, Gabrielle Euvino, and many others whose scholarship and wisdom enriched my thought process. I thank Colette Dowling; Alisa Pearson; Sonia Shah; Faith Gimzek; my sister, Kira Copperman; and my parents, Arthur and Barbara Phillips, for reading and commenting on chapters and drafts. I also thank my brother, Marc Phillips, for his humor and support.

Laney Salisbury read and critiqued excerpts, drafts, and ramblings over the years it took to write this book. More important, she reassured me, with the compassion and understanding that can come only from a fellow writer, when I became too overwrought about writing and life in general. She and Beth Reicheld gave me steady moral support and friendship, as did my SUNY New Paltz colleagues Patricia Sullivan, Howie Good, and Gregg Bray.

I thank my husband, Bill Mead, who has championed this project from its beginnings. And why wouldn't he? He's the noble gentleman who showed me what good love was—and he still does. As an artist, he understands the necessity of perseverance and focus. The house he built for our family includes a spacious office for me with a lovely view, the best place I could imagine to write this book.

I thank our daughter, Clara Mead, whose self-confidence and verve inspire me daily.

Finally, I thank the women and men who generously granted me in-depth interviews for this book. I am honored that you shared my belief that your stories will help others as they work through the challenges of unrequited love.

Notes

Introduction: The Unwanted Woman

3   **I surveyed more than 260 women online:** The online survey was launched on May 1, 2010. Results were retrieved on March 19, 2014, at which point the survey had 261 complete responses. I have used the survey during the writing of *Unrequited* not as a scientific measure of women's experiences of unrequited love but as a way to get a general sense of the range of women's experiences. I also used it to find women to interview. The survey was anonymous, but respondents had the option to give their contact information so they could be contacted for an interview. See http://www.lisaaphillips.com/survey/index.php?sid=24932&lang=en.

4   **to hurt the person who's rejecting them:** In a study that used functional magnetic resonance imaging (fMRI) to study ten women and men who had recently been rejected by a partner but reported they were still "intensely in love," all participants responded that they thought about their rejecter more than 85 percent of the time. The participants also reported "signs of lack of emotional control," including inappropriate phoning, writing, or emailing; pleading to get back together; long bouts of crying; drinking too much; and/or "making dramatic entrances and exits into the rejecter's home, place of work or social space" to express their feelings. Helen E. Fisher, Lucy L. Brown, Arthur Aron, Greg Strong, and Debra Mashek, "Reward, Addiction, and Emotion Regulation Systems

Associated with Rejection in Love," *Journal of Neurophysiology* 104 (2010): 51–52.

4   **93 percent of respondents had been rejected by someone they passionately loved:** Roy F. Baumeister and Sara R. Wotman surveyed upper-level college students about the frequency of their experiences of unrequited love. They found that by their early twenties, nearly everyone has had at least one experience on each side of unrequited love. Only one person out of every twenty said they had never had an unrequited-love experience. Roy F. Baumeister and Sara R. Wotman, *Breaking Hearts: The Two Sides of Unrequited Love* (New York: Guilford Press, 1992).

4   **there is no clear evidence that one sex is more vulnerable to it than the other:** Baumeister and Wotman's research in *Breaking Hearts* indicated that women were somewhat more likely to be in the rejecter role than the aspiring-lover role. Dorothy Tennov's research in *Love and Limerence* showed that more women than men reported they either "have been very depressed about a love affair" or thought they would "never get over" a broken relationship. See Baumeister and Wotman, *Breaking Hearts*, 12, and Dorothy Tennov, *Love and Limerence: The Experience of Being in Love* (Lanham, MD: Scarborough House, 1999).

4   **The median age of marriage is rising:** According to U.S. census data the median age of first marriage in 2010 was twenty-six for women and twenty-eight for men. In 1950, it was twenty for women and twenty-two for men. See "Median Age of First Marriage by Sex: 1890–2010," U.S. Decennial Census (1890–2000), http://www.census.gov/hhes/socdemo/marriage/data/acs/ElliottetalPAA2012figs.pdf.

4   **at last count, just 51 percent of adults eighteen and older are married:** In 1960, 72 percent of adults age eighteen and older were married. By 2010, 51 percent were. See "Barely Half of U.S. Adults Are Married—a Record Low," Pew Research Center, December 14, 2011, http://www.pewsocialtrends.org/2011/.

5   **Face the fact that he's "just not that into you" and forget about him ASAP:** "You're going to have to feel the pain, you're going to have to go through it, and then you're going to have to get over it" is the one-sentence prescription for moving on at the end of

He's Just Not That Into You, a book that goes into great detail about how to tell when a man is behaving in a way that indicates there's no hope for a relationship. Greg Behrendt and Liz Tuccillo, *He's Just Not That Into You* (New York: Simon & Schuster, 2004), 152.

6   **the couple married:** Sarah Lacy, *Once You're Lucky, Twice You're Good: The Rebirth of Silicon Valley and the Rise of Web 2.0* (New York: Gotham, 2009), 162.

6   **the expression has endured as slang for jealous exes and over-zealous aspiring lovers:** Some examples from Twitter: "She's going to find your bunny and boil it sister!"; "I'm sorry I trophied your twittercrush. Please don't boil my bunny." Accessed January 24, 2014, from a word search of "bunny boil" on www.twitter.com.

6   **Alex—the "most hated woman in America," according to one tabloid cover:** Susan Faludi, *Backlash* (New York: Crown, 1991), 117.

7   **wrapped in oilskin next to his heart:** The nineteenth-century explorer Henry Morton Stanley carried a photograph of his beloved, a seventeen-year-old American named Alice Pike, in such a fashion on a three-year expedition to explore the great lakes of central Africa. He named the boat he used *Lady Alice.* In love letters, he called her "my dream, my stay, my hope, and my beacon" and believed she would marry him. He returned to civilization only to learn from his publisher that she had gotten married to another man. Yet the idea of Alice had sustained him through bouts of disease, near starvation, confrontations with cannibals, and other hazards. His story is an example of the power of distraction—what Stanley called "self-forgetfulness"—to foster will-power. Roy F. Baumeister and John Tierney, *Willpower: Rediscovering the Greatest Human Strength* (New York: Penguin, 2011), 160–61.

7   **led to the passage of anti-stalking laws throughout the country:** Robert John Bardo, a nineteen-year-old unemployed fast-food worker, carried a publicity photo of Rebecca Schaeffer everywhere, called her agent several times, and sent her fan mail. He killed her after getting her address from the California Department of Motor Vehicles. That same year (1989), five Orange County, California, women were killed in a six-week period by former husbands or boyfriends after courts had issued restraining orders against the men to prevent harassment. California enacted the nation's first anti-stalking law in 1990. By the mid-1990s,

all the other states had followed suit. See Robert N. Miller, "Stalk Talk: A First Look at Anti-Stalking Legislation," *Washington and Lee Law Review* 50 (1991): 1,303–04.

8   **because men should be protecting women from harm:** Richard B. Felson, "Chivalry," *Violence and Gender Reexamined* (Washington, D.C.: American Psychological Association, 2002).

9   **Women are far more likely to be the *victims* of stalking than the perpetrators:** The National Intimate Partner and Sexual Violence Survey reports that one in six women (16.2 percent) and one in nineteen men (5.2 percent) in the United States have experienced stalking victimization at some point during their lifetime. Stalking victimization was defined as "a pattern of harassing or threatening tactics used by a perpetrator that is both unwanted and causes fear or safety concerns in the victim," similar to the definition used in most state anti-stalking statutes. Two thirds of the female victims (66.2 percent) reported stalking by a current or former intimate partner, and nearly one quarter (24 percent) reported stalking by an acquaintance. Approximately four out of ten male stalking victims (41.4 percent) reported they had been stalked by an intimate partner, and 40 percent had been stalked by an acquaintance. The NIPSV is an ongoing, nationally representative random-digit dial-telephone survey that gathers information about sexual violence, stalking, and intimate-partner violence among English- and Spanish-speaking women and men in the United States. The survey is conducted by the Centers for Disease Control's National Center for Injury Prevention and Control, with the support of the National Institute of Justice and the Department of Defense. M. C. Black et al, *The National Intimate Partner and Sexual Violence Survey: 2010 Summary Report* (Atlanta, GA: National Center for Injury Prevention and Control, Centers for Disease Control and Prevention), 29–33, http://www.cdc.gov/ViolencePrevention/pdf/NISVS_Report2010-a.pdf.

9   **more than one out of ten stalkers is female:** In a study of 1,005 stalking cases gathered from law enforcement, prosecutorial, and entertainment corporate security files, 14.2 percent were female. Six percent of the sample were "prior intimate stalkers," the category most relevant to this book. Stalking behavior was defined as "two or more

unwanted contacts by a subject toward a target that created a reasonable fear in that target." Two other community-based studies of stalking victimization found that 12 to 13 percent of stalkers were female. J. Reid Meloy, Kris Mohandie, and Mila Green. "The Female Stalker," *Behavioral Sciences and the Law* 29 (March/April 2011): 240–54.

9   **"obsessive relational intrusion" (ORI):** For an extensive discussion of ORI, see Brian H. Spitzberg and William R. Cupach, "What Mad Pursuit?: Obsessive Relational Intrusion and Stalking Related Phenomena," *Aggression and Violent Behavior* 8 (2003): 345–75.

9   **that causes the target to fear for his or her safety:** See Reid J. Meloy, ed., *The Psychology of Stalking: Clinical and Forensic Perspectives* (San Diego: Academic Press, 1998), 2.

10   **They're perceived as responsible for being stalked:** Stefanie Ashton Wigman, "Male Victims of Former-Intimate Stalking: A Selected Review," *International Journal of Men's Health* 8 (2009): 108–12.

11   **"Alec is a sicko. Everyone knows it":** Tom Hays, "Genevieve Sabourin, Canadian Actress Accused of Stalking Alec Baldwin, Arrested in Manhattan," *Huffington Post*, November 27, 2012, http://www .huffingtonpost.com/2012/11/28/genevieve-sabourin_n_2203706. html.

12   **"made me into a fighter":** Neil Strauss, "The Broken Heart and Violent Fantasies of Lady Gaga," *Rolling Stone*, July 8, 2010, http://www .rollingstone.com/music/news/the-broken-heart-and-violent-fantasies-of-lady-gaga-20100708.

1: Do You Love Me?

16   **they are clearly meant for each other:** Several readers of the 1905 best seller *The House of Mirth* protested the novel's ending because they thought Lawrence should have married (and thus saved) Lily. According to a story in *The Detroit News*, one fan reprimanded Wharton on the street for Lily Bart's suicide. Amy L. Blair, "Misreading *The House of Mirth*," *American Literature*, 76 (March 2004): 149–75.

17   **In ancient Egypt:** The hieroglyphic sign for love was a hoe, a mouth, and a man with a hand in his mouth. M. Abdel-Kader Hatem, *Life in Ancient Egypt* (Los Angeles: Gateway Publishers, 1976).

19   **suffer the misery of rejection:** A poem by the twelfth-century French troubadour Bernart de Ventadorn ends in the fashion typical of the time: "I go away, wretched, I know not where / I will withdraw from singing and renounce it / And I hide myself from joy and love."

19   **see her naked body without touching it:** Diane Ackerman, *A Natural History of Love* (New York: Random House, 1994), 48–54.

19   **Courtly love gave the knight a higher purpose in life:** "Because courtly love was extramarital, it was an accomplishment based on the desire to control the impatience of instinct, on the successful passing of a series of initiatory tests and finally on the discovery, thanks to the *dame*, of the lady, or a world of spiritual values." Danielle Jacquart, Claude Thomasett, and Matthew Adamson, *Sexuality and Medicine in the Middle Ages* (Princeton, NJ: Princeton University Press, 1998), 95.

20   **sublimated his desire into prowess on the battlefield:** Barbara Tuchman, *A Distant Mirror: The Calamitous 14th Century* (New York: Random House, 1987), 66–68.

20   **ascended with her to heaven:** Quotations are from Dante Alighieri, *La Vita Nuova* (New York: Penguin Books, 2004).

20   **many love sonnets he would compose in her honor:** Ibid., 5.

21   **He preferred instead to write "words of praise":** Dante recounts a conversation with "a group of ladies, who were aware of my feelings." They press him to explain "What is the point of your love for your lady since you are unable to endure her presence?" He explains that because Beatrice no longer greets him when she sees him, he has decided to "place his joy in something which cannot fail me," which he explains as "words which praise my lady"—his poetry. Ibid., 24.

21   **"The gaze is not upon the woman:** R. Howard Bloch, *Medieval Misogyny and the Invention of Western Romantic Love* (Chicago: University of Chicago Press, 1992), 149.

21   **more than a means to gain property and perpetuate a bloodline:** "Women's status improved, less for her own sake than as the inspirer of male glory, a higher function than being merely a sexual object, a breeder of children, or a conveyor of property." See Tuchman, *A Distant Mirror*, 67.

22   **she arranges for her funeral barge to greet him:** MaryLynn Saul, "Courtly Love and Patriarchal Marriage Practice in Malory's *Le Morte d'Arthur*" in *Fifteenth-Century Studies* 24 (1998): 55–56.

22   **He had a reputation for being sexually impotent:** Matthew Josephson, in his biography of Stendhal, recounts an evening in Paris in 1921 when Stendhal went to a brothel with friends for an encounter with a prostitute whose beauty was celebrated. Consumed with love for Mathilde Dembowski, he was too sad to go through with the act, and his friends mocked him. *Stendhal or The Pursuit of Happiness* (New York: Doubleday & Company, Inc., 1946), 268–69.

22   **the protagonists in his novels:** When the protagonist of *Lucien Leuwen* rides under the window of the beautiful Mme. de Chasteller, he falls off his horse; Fabrizio in *The Charterhouse of Parma* struggles with his attraction to his aunt Gina, who loves him passionately.

23   **"the deep sorrow caused me by my defeats":** Stendhal, *The Life of Henry Brulard,* trans. Catherine Alison Phillips (New York: Alfred A. Knopf, 1939), 5.

24   **"Everything is new, everything is alive:** Stendhal, *On Love*, trans. Philip Sidney Woolf and Cecil N. Sidney Woolf (Mount Vernon, NY: Peter Pauper Press, 1853), 201.

24   **"The girl is a fool; the man a tragic hero":** Christina Nehring, *A Vindication of Love: Reclaiming Romance for the Twenty-first Century* (New York: Harper, 2009), 24–25.

24   **what he perceived as a woman's ultimate power:** "Should not a woman's true pride reside in the power of the feelings she inspired?" Stendhal, *On Love*, 71.

25   **she has since remarried:** Ellen Fein separated from her first husband in 2000, just as *The Rules for Marriage: Time-Tested Secrets for Making Your Marriage Work* was being shipped to bookstores. She tried to sue her cosmetic dentist for ruining her teeth and her marriage. She remarried in 2008. She told *The New York Times* that she'd found her new husband by following *The Rules.* See Lois Smith Brady, "Vows: Ellen Fein and Lance Houpt," *The New York Times*, August 10, 2008, ST13.

25   **the main arguments . . . have had remarkable staying power:** At this writing, the latest incarnation of the *Rules* juggernaut is *Not Your*

Mother's Rules: The New Secrets for Dating (The Rules) by Ellen Fein and Sherrie Schneider (New York: Grand Central, 2013). The original book in the series, *The Rules™: Time-Tested Secrets for Capturing the Heart of Mr. Right*, was published by the same authors with Warner Books in 1995.

29 **organizes our lives, thoughts, and actions:** This idea comes from Robert Michael's writings on political passions in student rebels of the late 1960s but is certainly relevant to romantic passion: "From a psychological point of view, passion is quite different from patterns of either thought or action because, unlike these, it cannot be compartmentalized or isolated from other personality functions. True passion organizes an individual's life, his every thought and action, and allows no compromise. It is, to borrow a phrase, 'nonnegotiable.'" See Milton Viederman's description of Robert Michael's work in "The Nature of Passionate Love" in *Passionate Attachments: Thinking About Love*, edited by Willard Gaylin, M.D., and Ethel Person, M.D. (New York: Free Press, 1988), 4.

30 **a "future state of perfect happiness":** Sharon Brehm, "Passionate Love" in R. A. Sternberg and M. Barnes, eds., *The Psychology of Love* (New Haven, CT: Yale University Press), 253.

30 **across world cultures and religions:** Semir Zeki, *Splendors and Miseries of the Brain: Love, Creativity, and the Quest for Human Happiness* (West Sussex, UK: John Wiley & Sons, 2009), Kindle edition, location 2703.

37 **be-all and end-all of intimacy:** Katherine's unrequited loves bring to mind Laura Kipnis's argument against marital fidelity: "Sometimes desire just won't take no for an answer, particularly when some beguiling and potentially available love-object hovers into your sight lines, making you feel what you'd forgotten how to feel, which is *alive*, even though you're supposed to be channeling all such affective capacities into the 'appropriate' venues, and everything (Social Stability! The National Fabric! Being a Good Person!) hinges on making sure that you do. But renunciation chafes, particularly when the quantities demanded begin to exceed the amount of gratification achieved." *Against Love: A Polemic* (New York: Pantheon, 2003), 44.

38 **"the enchanted gardens of the imagination":** Stendhal, *On Love*, 53.

2: Holding Out

40 **"seal with which lovers plight their troth"**: William J. Fielding, *Strange Customs of Courtship and Marriage* (New York: New Home Library, 1942), 55.

44 **"There's a special place in hell"**: Swift has also been criticized for buying a house near the Kennedy compound in Cape Cod during her brief relationship with Conor Kennedy (which she's since sold) and making veiled barbs at ex-boyfriend Harry Styles at the 2013 VMA awards. See Nancy Jo Sales, "Taylor Swift's Telltale Heart," *Vanity Fair*, April 2013, 11; Andrew Gruttadaro, "Taylor Swift Disses Harry Styles While Accepting her VMA Award," Hollywoodlife. com, August 25, 2013, http://hollywoodlife.com/2013/08/25/harry-styles-taylor-swift-diss-vmas-speech/; and Rachel McRady, "Tina Fey Slams Taylor Swift," *Us Weekly*, January 13, 2014, http://www .usmagazine.com/celebrity-news/news/tina-fey-slams-taylor-swift-while-congratulating-amy-poehler-theres-a-special-place in hell-for-you-2014131.

46 **how much she wanted him back:** "Platonic friendship makes the issue of persistence especially painful. The would-be lover may agree to remain 'just friends,' but the feelings do not necessarily go away, and the continued contact provides a constant reminder and stimulus to the desire." Baumeister and Wotman, *Breaking Hearts*, 164.

46 **whatever signs she can grab on to:** Ibid., 158–9.

46 **because sometimes they do:** Hillary J. Morgan and Phillip R. Shaver, "Attachment Processes and Commitment to Romantic Relationships," in *Handbook of Interpersonal Commitment and Relationship Stability*, eds. Jeffrey M. Adamas and Warren H. Jones (New York: Kluwer Academic/Plenum Publishers, 1999), 119.

47 **didn't want me to contact the object of her longing:** I, like other writers and researchers who have examined unrequited love, face the impossibility of getting both sides of the story. Interview subjects— unrequited lovers and rejecters alike—rarely agree to identify the people they're talking about, much less consent to let you contact them.

47 **no, this isn't going to work:** The common reluctance to transmit bad news to people has been called the "mum effect." Roy F.

Baumeister et al, "Unrequited Love: On Heartbreak, Anger, Guilt, Scriptlessness, and Humiliation," *Journal of Personality and Social Psychology* 64 (1993): 377–94. See also Abraham Tesser and Sidney Rosen, "The Reluctance to Transmit Bad News," *Advances in Experimental Social Psychology*, ed. L. Berkowitz (San Diego, CA: Academic Press, 1975), 193–232.

48   **similar neural mechanisms are at work in both kinds of love:** Frank Tallis, *Love Sick: Love as a Mental Illness* (New York: Thunder's Mouth Press, 2004), 251–52.

48   **turning his back on this most basic human desire:** "Attachment theory portrays human beings as organisms craving to form social bonds with each other, and so it is surprising to find a person rejecting attachment." Baumeister et al, *Breaking Hearts*, 34.

49   **toying with a vulnerable woman:** "One of the gender differences that stood out is the higher appetite for sex among men, especially casual sex. Having someone with a crush on you is an opportunity for that. Whether knowingly exploiting the difference or just thinking, great, I get to have sex—men are drawn into that. Whereas if the man is attracted to the woman and she doesn't reciprocate, she's not going to think having sex with him is all that appealing." Roy Baumeister, in-person interview, October 25, 2013.

49   **Janey's ex is wrong for leading her on:** "To show attraction to another and then withdraw it is regarded as inconsistent, teasing, unfair. The common term is 'leading the person on,' and it violates the norms for appropriate treatment of other people." Baumeister and Wotman, *Breaking Hearts*, 141–42.

49   **can have the same power:** Baumeister and Wotman note that their research subjects can sustain a "self-deceptive persistence" despite "multiple and clear messages of rejection" when a beloved's interest fades. Baumeister and Wotman, *Breaking Hearts*, 159.

49   **arranged marriages in Western culture:** Charles Lindholm describes the early-nineteenth-century shift from arranged marriage to marriages of choice as stemming from the rise of the bourgeoisie. The bourgeois individual's life was increasingly divided between home and the workplace, which led to the rise of individualism and intimate personal relationships. "Increased personal choice and individuality,

along with a new emphasis on intimacy, meant that marriage was now constituted not by interest or duty, as in previous generations, but by the mutual idealization of romantic love. Love marriage has usually been portrayed by sociologists . . . as a necessary functional aid to the integration of a fragmented modern world." Charles Lindholm, "The Future of Love," in *Romantic Love and Sexual Behavior: Perspectives from the Social Sciences*, ed. Victor C. Munck (Westport, CT: Praeger, 1998), 18.

50 **Women responded by granting them time:** Karen Lystra, *Searching the Heart: Women, Men, and Romantic Love in Nineteenth-Century America* (New York: Oxford University Press, 1989), 186–87.

50 **kissing and heavy petting:** "Some indeterminate level of sexual expression and satisfaction was acceptable in Victorian courtships when individuals were in love and the expectation of marriage was strong. . . . Imbued with romantic love, sex was seen as an act of self-disclosure, not so much in the sense of revealing one's body as one's essential identity. Sex was identified with the inner life and was perceived as part of the privileged revelation of an 'authentic' self. Properly sanctioned by love, sexual expressions were read as symbolic communications of one's real and truest self, part of the hidden essence of the individual." Ibid., 59.

50 **the initials of the boys they'd broken up with:** "In earlier days going steady had been more like the old-fashioned 'keeping steady company'. It was a step along the path to marriage, even if many steady couples parted company before they reached their destination. By the early 1950s, going steady had acquired a totally different meaning. It was no longer the way a marriageable couple signaled their deepening intentions. Instead, going steady was something twelve-year-olds could do, something most fifteen-year-olds did. Few steady couples expected to marry each other (especially the twelve-year-olds), but, for the duration, they acted *as if* they were married. Going steady had become a sort of play-marriage, a mimicry of the actual marriage of their slightly older peers." Beth L. Baily, *From Front Porch to Back Seat: Courtship in Twentieth-Century America* (Baltimore: Johns Hopkins University Press, 1988), 49–52.

50 **As late as 1970:** Barbara Whitehead, *Why There Are No Good Men Left: The Romantic Plight of the New Single Woman* (New York: Broadway Books, 2003), 11–13.

51 **lost in the shuffle is "any coherent set of widely accepted practices or conventions":** Ibid., 13–14.

51 **too many varieties of jam:** Barry Schwartz, *The Paradox of Choice: Why More Is Less* (New York: Ecco Press, 2003), 19.

51 **too many prospects in a speed-dating session:** Sander van der Linden, "Speed Dating and Decision-Making: Why Less Is More," June 7, 2011, http://www.scientificamerican.com/article.cfm?id=speed-dating-decision-making-why-less-is-more.

51 **for men, who can wait longer:** This issue, of course, is far more complicated. What's actually happening is a complex sociological dynamic that relates to delayed marriage and childbearing, decreasing marriage rates, women's increased educational and professional accomplishments, and the decrease in men's educational attainment and job prospects. For a comprehensive discussion, see Kate Bolick's November 2011 *Atlantic* article "All the Single Ladies" and Hanna Rosin's *The End of Men* (New York: Riverhead, 2012).

53 *Why didn't you call me?*: Macy Gray, "Why Didn't You Call Me," on *On How Life Is*, Epic Records, 1999.

53 **He needs space:** "The rejecter hopes that a few unreturned phone calls would be sufficient to convey to the would-be lover that the love is doomed. The would-be lover wants to see each unreturned phone call as accident, oversight, inconvenience, indeed as anything except as a sign of lack of interest." Baumeister and Wotman, *Breaking Hearts*, 140.

53 **an unstated cost-benefit calculation:** Miriam J. Rodin, "Non-Engagement, Failure to Engage, Disengagement," in *Personal Relationships 4: Dissolving Personal Relationships*, ed. Steve Duck (New York: Academic Press, 1982), 38–39.

54 **bestowing value isn't evidence-based:** The concepts of appraisal and bestowal, developed by Irving Singer, are discussed in *Romantic Love* by Susan S. Hendrick and Clyde Hendrick (Newbury Park, CA: Sage Publications, Inc., 1992), 31–34.

54 **falling in love is something they can't control:** Morgan and Shaver, "Attachment Process," 109.

57 **we'll put in the effort:** William R. Cupach and Brian H. Spitzberg, *The Dark Side of Relationship Pursuit* (Mahwah, NJ: Lawrence Erlbaum Associates, Inc., 2004), 100.

57   **the more they valued the goal of having a relationship:** The Arons describe unreciprocated love as a "motivational paradox." Typically, people love because they believe they will benefit from an intimate relationship, for example, the love the partner will give them. "Thus, it is paradoxical that one should love a person when it is known that the other does not love the self." Arthur Aron, Elaine N. Aron, and Joselyn Allen, "Motivations for Unreciprocated Love," *Personality and Social Psychology Bulletin* 24 (1998): 787.

58   **lower goals are supposed to be flexible and substitutable:** See Cupach and Spitzberg, *The Dark Side of Relationship Pursuit*, 98–101.

3: Erotic Melancholy

67   **Iustus's wife was besotted with Plyades:** Galen, *On Prognosis*, trans. Vivian Nutton (Berlin: Akademie-Verlag, 1979), http://cmg.bbaw.de/epubl/online/cmg_05_08_01.html, 100-102.

67   **a woman being diagnosed with lovesickness:** Mary Frances Wack, *Lovesickness in the Middle Ages: The Viaticum and Its Commentaries* (Philadelphia: University of Pennsylvania Press, 1990), 9.

68   **causing her physical symptoms:** Tallis, *Love Sick*, 13.

68   **perishes as his ship sails away:** Ackerman, *A Natural History of Love*, 31–39.

69   **would be adulterous, disreputable, and illegal:** Wack, *Lovesickness in the Middle Ages*, 9–10.

69   **to ever marry their paramours:** Jérôme Carcopino, *Daily Life in Ancient Rome: The People and the City at the Height of the Empire*, 2nd ed. (New Haven: Yale University Press, 2003), 94.

69   **the standard cure for lovesickness:** Oribasius, drawing on the work of Rufus of Ephesus, a famous physician of the late empire, recommended therapeutic intercourse for melancholy. Later, Arabic and European physicians promoted therapeutic intercourse as a cure for obsessive love. See Wack, *Lovesickness in the Middle Ages*, 10.

69   **but these were options available only to men:** Carol Thomas Neely, *Distracted Subjects: Madness and Gender in Shakespeare and Early Modern Culture* (Ithaca, NY: Cornell University Press, 2004), 102.

70   **Antiochus was instantly cured:** The story of Stratonice and Antiochus is from the "Life of Demetrius" by Plutarch in *Plutarch's Lives* (New York and Pittsburgh: Colonia Company Ltd., 1905), 134–36. Excerpt reprinted at http://classicpersuasion.org/pw/sappho/stratoni.htm.

70   **the buildup of sperma:** "The cure for love is frequent coitus," proclaimed the ninth-century physician Muhammad al-Razi, who was echoed by Ibn al-Jazzar, Avicenna, and a number of other Arabic practitioners. Wack, *Lovesickness in the Middle Ages*, 11.

70   **Arabic medical handbooks into Latin:** Ibid., xiii.

70   **a term that translates as "heroic love":** Jacques Ferrand, *A Treatise on Lovesickness*, trans. and ed. Donald A. Beecher and Massimo Ciavolella (Syracuse, NY: Syracuse University Press, 1990), 75.

71   **primarily affecting noblemen:** Wack points out that even though physicians in the early Middle Ages held that *amor hereos* was a disease of noblemen, female vulnerability to the condition was evident in the literature of the time. Lisa, an apothecary's daughter, in Chapter X of Boccaccio's *Decameron*, falls in obsessive unrequited love with King Peter of Aragon. She wastes away "like snow in the rays of the sun." See Wack, *Lovesickness in the Middle Ages*, 109.

71   **Discussions of "erotic melancholy":** Peter of Spain wrote extensively about the differences between male and female sexual physiology and lovesickness, also called "erotic melancholy," in his *Questions on the Viaticum*. He concluded that while men may be harder to cure because they suffer more intensely, women fall prey to the disease more often. Historian Mary Wack speculates that his interest in women stemmed from the fact that more women, particularly well-to-do ones, were showing up for treatment. Wack, *Lovesickness in the Middle Ages*, 123.

71   **less likely to interfere with rationality:** Ferrand, *A Treatise on Lovesickness*, 312.

72   **The prospect of sexual humiliation:** Ferrand, *A Treatise on Lovesickness*, 264.

72   **before she has brushed her hair and primped for the day:** Danielle Jacquart and Claude Thomasset, *Sexuality and Medicine in the*

Middle Ages, trans. Matthew Adamson (Princeton, NJ: Princeton University Press, 1988), 85.

72 **"what you love so much is nothing but vileness and filth":** Ferrand, *A Treatise on Lovesickness*, 318.

73 **Women who were attracted to other women:** Cheshire Calhoun, "Family Outlaws: Rethinking the Connections Between Feminism, Lesbianism, and the Family," in *Feminism and Families (Thinking Gender)*, ed. Hilde Lindemann Nelson (London: Routledge, 1997), 139.

74 **Tait took his place in the marital bed:** For a detailed account of Mary Sidgwick Benson's life, see *The Impossible Life of Mary Benson: The Extraordinary Story of a Victorian Wife* (New York: Atlantic Books, 2012).

74 **under the 1857 law:** The 1857 Matrimonial Causes Act made divorce a civil matter and established the Court of Divorce and Matrimonial Causes to decide divorce cases. Before then, a divorce could be granted only by an act of Parliament, a burdensome and expensive process that made divorce prohibitive for the middle class. See the introduction and prologue to *Mrs. Robinson's Disgrace: the Private Diary of a Victorian Lady* by Kate Summerscale (New York: Bloomsbury, 2012); the subsequent summary of the Robinson case and Isabella Robinson's life is based on details from this book.

76 **the place where we sought ecstasy, contentment, and awe:** See Tallis, *Love Sick*, 106. Sociologist Anthony Giddens also argues that modern love is "unique in its 'one and only' and 'forever' qualities, and in its insistence on the beloved as the source of a mystical sense of completion for the love. Overwhelming sexual desire, predominant in the passionate love of earlier social worlds, has become etherealized in romantic attraction and integrated into a larger narrative of a shared life course made meaningful by love." Lindholm, *The Future of Love*, 18.

76 **the wild state the Romantic era so venerated:** Tennov, *Love and Limerence*, 175–79.

81 **"relationship obsessive-compulsive disorder":** See Guy Doron, M. Mizrahi, O. Szepsenwol, D. Derby, "Right or Flawed: Relationships Obsessions and Sexual Satisfaction," *The Journal of Sexual Medicine* (2014). doi: 10.111/jsm.12616.

82   **building a body of research:** See Albert Wakin and Duyen B. Vo, "Love-Variant: The Wakin-Vo I.D.R. Model of Limerence," at http://www.persons.org.uk/ptb/persons/pil/pil2/wakinvo%20paper.pdf.

82   **gave them a shock of recognition:** Telephone interview with Albert Wakin, October 14, 2011.

82   **"a perfectly horrible addiction when it's going poorly":** This quote, which occurs in some form in several of Fisher's recent publications on love, is taken from her February 2008 TED talk, found at http://www.ted.com/talks/helen_fisher_studies_the_brain_in_love.

83   **Both groups had serotonin levels 40 percent lower than the control group:** Donna Marazziti, H. S. Akiskal, A. Rossi, G. B. Cassano, "Alternation of the Platelet Serotonin Transporter in Romantic Love," *Psychological Medicine* 29 (1999): 741–45.

83   **what they can do to get back the rejecter:** My description of the research on the impact of romantic rejection is based on the following sources: Helen E. Fisher et al, "Reward, Addiction, and Emotional Regulation Systems Associated With Rejection in Love," 51–60; Fisher's February 2008 TED talk; and a website Fisher and her colleague, neuroscientist Lucy Brown, put together on their research on love: http://theanatomyoflove.com/.

84   **"New Love: A Short Shelf Life":** Sonia Lyubomirsky, "New Love: A Short Shelf Life," *The New York Times*, December 1, 2012, http://www.nytimes.com/2012/12/02/opinion/sunday/new-love-a-short-shelf-life.html.

84   **"Anti-Love Drug May Be Ticket to Bliss":** John Tierney, "Anti-Love Drug May Be Ticket to Bliss," *The New York Times*, January 12, 2009, http://www.nytimes.com/2009/01/13/science/13tier.html?_r=0.

84   **not overvalue passion and romance:** Tallis, *Love Sick*, 257–88.

84   **rival or exceed those of couples in marriages of choice:** Jayamala Madathil and James M. Benschoff, "Importance of Marital Characteristics and Marital Satisfaction: A Comparison of Asian Indians in Arranged Marriages and Americans in Marriages of Choice," *The Family Journal* 16 (July 2008): 222–30.

85   **a significant contrast to the historical examples:** Since I first spoke with Samara (her real name, which she requested I use) in 2011,

she wrote and published a self-help book about getting over romantic rejection. The book includes some of the material she shared with me. See Samara O'Shea, *Loves Me . . . Not: How to Survive (and Thrive!) in the Face of Unrequited Love* (New York: February Books, 2014).

85   **"chemical breakup" remedies:** Brian D. Earp, Olga A. Wudarczyk, Anders Sandberg, and Julian Savulescu, "If I Could Just Stop Loving You: Anti-love Biotechnology and the Ethics of a Chemical Breakup," *American Journal of Bioethics* 13 (2013): 17.

86   **strict rules on masturbation and sexual intercourse:** Yair Ettinger, "Rabbi's Little Helper," *Haaretz*, April 6, 2012, http://www .haaretz.com/weekend/week-s-end/rabbi-s-little-helper-1.422985.

86   **antidepressants in order to endure their spouses:** Louisa Kamps, "The Couple Who Medicates Together," *Elle*, April 18, 2012, http:// www.elle.com/life-love/sex-relationships/the-couple-who-medicates- together-654677.

86   **sufferers are under the delusion:** Historically, as I've discussed, erotomania referred generally to obsessive unrequited love or excessive sexual desire. In the present-day definition of the term, people with erotomania, a type of delusional disorder also known as de Clérambault's syndrome, have an unshakable belief that another person—often a celebrity or someone of higher social status—is in love with them. Erotomania, a rare condition diagnosed more often in women than in men, is interesting in that it seems a distorted, pathological manifestation of the resistance that more everyday forms of unrequited love can entail: This love will break down divides and transport me to a better world. But because erotomania is a delusion often accompanying psychosis, I'm reluctant to tie the qualities of the disorder too closely with my discussion of more common experiences of unrequited love. The metaphorical resonances of erotomania are brilliantly explored in Ian McEwan's 1997 novel, *Enduring Love*; see also Robert Lloyd-Goldstein, "De Clérambault On-Line: A Survey of Erotomania and Stalking from the Old World to the World Wide Web" in *The Psychology of Stalking: Clinical and Forensic Perspectives*, ed. J. Reid Meloy (San Diego: Academic Press, 1998). For a discussion of borderline personality disorder, a condition the *DSM-IV* describes as characterized by "a pattern of

unstable and intense interpersonal relationships" and "frantic efforts to avoid real or imagined abandonment," see Randy A. Sansone and Lori A. Sansone, "Fatal Attraction Syndrome: Stalking Behavior and Borderline Personality," *Psychiatry* 7 (May 2010): 42–46.

86 **forces that spur reproduction and make the human experience richer, albeit more challenging and complex:** "Because there is a positive relationship between dopamine (associated with romantic love) and testosterone (linked to sexual desire and arousal) and because there is a negative relationship between serotonin and these catecholamines and the androgens, serotonin-enhancing antidepressants can also inhibit feelings of romantic love. Moreover, because serotonin-enhancing antidepressants have a negative impact on penile erection, sexual arousal, orgasm, and other evolved psychobiological courtship mechanisms, these drugs can also negatively affect one's ability to signal genetic and psychological fitness, assess and select potential mating partners, pursue preferred individuals, and maintain stable pair bonds." See Helen E. Fisher and J. Anderson Thomson, Jr., "Lust, Romance, Attachment: Do the Side Effects of Serotonin-Enhancing Antidepressants Jeopardize Romantic Love, Marriage, and Fertility?" in *Evolutionary Cognitive Neuroscience*, ed. Steven M. Platek et al (Cambridge, MA: MIT Press, 2006), 269–70.

87 **It's a meritocracy applied to personal life:** Adelle Waldman, *The Love Affairs of Nathaniel P.* (New York: Henry Holt and Co., 2013), 79.

91 **"dependence on him that often increases":** Emma Jung, *Animus and Anima* (Woodstock, CT: Spring Publications, Inc., 1957), 10.

4: Boy Chasers

95 **Testosterone . . . goes up in women and decreases in men:** Donatella Marazziti and Domenico Canale, "Hormonal Changes When Falling in Love," *Psychoneuroendocrinology* 29 (2004): 931–36.

95 **How this testosterone fluctuation affects our behavior hasn't been studied yet:** Marazziti and Canale wrote, "It is tempting to link the changes in testosterone levels to changes in behaviours, sexual at-

titudes or, perhaps, aggressive traits which move in different directions in the two sexes, however, apart from some anecdotal evidence, we have no data substantiating this, which would justify further research." See Marazziti and Canale, "Hormonal Changes When Falling in Love," 2004.

95 **"as if nature wants to eliminate what can be different in men and women":** "In Love We're Not So Different," *The Daily Mail*, accessed at http://www.dailymail.co.uk/femail/article-300871/In-love-different.html.

95 **an increase in positive emotions:** A 2008 study looked at levels of cortisol release in women described as doing "a high amount of relationship-focused thinking" compared to women who don't tend to think about relationships as much. The women who thought more about relationships had a higher increase in cortisol. See Timothy J. Loving, Erin E. Crockett, and Aubri A. Paxson, "Passionate Love and Relationship Thinkers: Experimental Evidence for Acute Cortisol Elevations in Women," *Psychoneuroendocrinology* 34 (2009): 939–46.

96 **the heat of desire:** Ferrand, *A Treatise on Lovesickness*, 230.

96 **cover and authority to successfully win over their love interests:** In the worldview of the Renaissance era, women were considered less rational than men and in need of male protection. Dressed as men, women could travel alone, bear arms, and interact with their beloveds with increased authority. In several of Shakespeare's plays, female characters dress as men to pursue the men they love and take some control over the courtship process. Examples include Julia in *The Two Gentlemen of Verona* and Viola in *Twelfth Night*. See Jean E. Howard, "Cross-dressing, the Theatre, and Gender Struggle in Early Modern England," *Shakespeare Quarterly* 1988 (39): 418–40.

96 **her redemptive self-sacrifice for Marius:** *Les Misérables* was published in 1862. Adèle left for Halifax in 1863.

97 **where she would live for the rest of her life:** Adèle's affect after her return has been described by Hugo biographer Graham Robb as "emotionless"; she would talk to voices in her head. Graham Robb, *Victor Hugo* (New York: W. W. Norton, 1997), 475.

98   **enter places otherwise forbidden to women:** My description of Adèle Hugo's life is based on two sources: Robb's *Victor Hugo* and Leslie Smith Dow, *Adèle Hugo: La Misérable* (Fredericton, NB: Goose Lane Editions, 1993).

99   **"she is in a long-term relationship with exactly *none* of the men she has pursued!":** Tracy McMillan, *Why You're Not Married . . . Yet: The Straight Talk You Need to Get the Relationship You Deserve* (Ballantine Books, 2013), 162.

100   **Straight women say they initiate about 40 percent of their relationships:** Catherine L. Clark, Phillip R. Shaver, and Matthew Abrahams, "Strategic Behaviors in Romantic Relationship Initiation," *Personality and Social Psychology Bulletin* 25 (1999), 713.

100   **tease information out of mutual friends:** Stacey L. Williams and Irene Hanson Frieze, "Courtship Behaviors, Relationship Violence, and Breakup Persistence in College Men and Women," *Psychology of Women Quarterly* 29 (2005), 252.

100   **women engage in pursuit behaviors at similar rates to men:** Results of these studies are published in the following articles: H. Colleen Sinclair and Irene Hanson Frieze, "Initial Courtship Behavior and Stalking: How Should We Draw the Line?," *Violence and Victims* 15, no. 1 (2000); Jennifer Langhinrichsen-Rohling et al, "Breaking Up Is Hard to Do: Unwanted Pursuit Behaviors Following the Dissolution of a Romantic Relationship," *Violence and Victims* 15, no. 1 (2000); Leila B. Dutton and Barbara A. Winstead, "Predicting Unwanted Pursuit: Attachment, Relationship Satisfaction, Relationship Alternatives, and Breakup Distress," *Journal of Social and Personal Relationships* 23 (2006): 565.

101   **while a man thrives on competition:** *Why You're Not Married . . . Yet* mingles evolutionary psychology with New Age gender essentialism: "The woman grounded in her Feminine understands that her investment in her egg is *way, way, way* bigger than the man's investment in his sperm. Guys are sperm factories . . . if you let someone fertilize the egg, that's gonna be eighteen-plus years of your life that you invest in that egg. *Of course* you need to be selective." See McMillan, *Why You're Not Married . . . Yet*, 70. Sherry Argov, the author of the "Bitches" series (*Why Men Marry Bitches, Why Men Love Bitches*),

also taps in to superficial evolutionary clichés: "Women need to understand that men love the 'thrill of the chase' and are highly competitive. They like racing cars, engaging in athletics, and hunting. They like to fix things, to figure things out, to pursue." See Sherry Argov, *Why Men Love Bitches: From Doormat to Dreamgirl* (Avon, MA: Adams Media, 2009), 26.

102 **to see if humans could survive trips to the moon:** Bergner also discusses a speed-dating study at Northwestern University that shows that eliminating even one minor gendered norm in courtship can have an impact on the male pursuer/female pursued paradigm. The study showed that when women were the "rotators" in a speed-dating scenario (they were the ones to get up and approach new prospects— speed-dating sessions almost always give that role to the man because it's "more chivalrous"), women were more likely to feel attracted to more of the men. Giving women the approach role "eradicated sex differences in romantic selectivity." The power to approach made women feel more confident and more likely to say they wanted to see the prospect again. Daniel Bergner, *What Do Women Want?: Adventures in the Science of Female Desire* (New York: Ecco Press, 2013), 43–66.

103 **Women outnumber men on college campuses nationwide:** Women get 57 percent of bachelor's degrees and 60 percent of master's degrees (at SUNY New Paltz, where the female-to-male ratio is 65 to 35, most of my journalism classes are less than a quarter male). Interestingly, attending a majority-female campus is linked to later motherhood—and increased professional success. A study by researchers led by University of Texas at San Antonio professor Kristina Durante found that the scarcer bachelors were in college, the greater the percentage of women who entered high-paying careers and delayed having children. Hans Villarica, "Study of the Day: Gender Gap in College Leads Women to Prioritize Work," *The Atlantic*, May 7, 2012, http://www.theatlantic.com/health/archive/2012/05/study-of-the-day-gender-gap-in-college-leads-women-to-prioritize-work/256795.

106 **Intense pursuit and expressions of need:** Evolutionary psychologist Marco Del Giudice hypothesizes that because males have less at stake, reproductively speaking, from sexual intercourse, males living under conditions of high environmental stress will show higher levels

of avoidance than females, which is part of a low-investment, low-commitment strategy. Anxiety, on the other hand, may be a way for females living under the same environmental conditions to secure and extract investment (attention and protection for themselves and their theoretical or real offspring) from both family members and sexual partners. Glenn Geher and Scott Barry Kaufman, *Mating Intelligence Unleashed: The Role of the Mind in Sex, Dating, and Love* (New York: Oxford University Press, 2013), 103.

107 **"pre-relationship" stalking as a strategy to win a mate:** See Joshua D. Duntley and David M. Buss, "The Evolution of Stalking," *Sex Roles* 66 (2012): 311–27.

107 **sexual infidelity, which could trick them:** See David M. Buss, *The Dangerous Passion: Why Jealousy Is as Necessary as Love and Sex* (New York: Free Press, 2000).

108 **engage in the world in a focused and secure way:** R. Chris Fraley and Phillip R. Shaver, "Adult Romantic Attachment: Theoretical Developments, Emerging Controversies, and Unanswered Questions," *Review of General Psychology* 4 (2000): 136–38.

108 **Men and women react to separation and loss:** There is an "emerging consensus among neurobiologists and social-personality psychologists that both parent-infant bonds and long-term couple relationships draw on the *same* attachment motivational system." Behavioral and psychological displays of bond formation, separation, and loss are similar in adults and children, and these similiarities are reflected in neurochemistry and neuroanatomy. Geher and Kaufman, *Mating Intelligence Unleashed*, 242.

108 **"protest response," activated when emotional attachments are ruptured:** Thomas Lewis, Fari Amini, and Richard Lannon, *A General Theory of Love* (New York: Random House, 2000), 75.

109 **Brain scans of men and women who have been rejected recently look similar:** Telephone interview with Arthur Aron on March 29, 2013.

109 **are less extreme than criminal stalking:** Kim S. Menard and Aaron L. Pincus, "Predicting Overt and Cyber Stalking Perpetration by Male and Female College Students," *Journal of Interpersonal Violence* 27 (2012): 2197.

109   **are more given to experiencing unrequited love:** Aron et al, "Motivations for Unreciprocated Love," 787.

109   **romantic rejection in both opposite-sex and same-sex scenarios:** See Cupach and Spitzberg, *The Dark Side of Relationship Pursuit*, 96–97, and Valerian J. Derlega et al, "Unwanted Pursuit in Same-Sex Relationships: Effects of Attachment Styles, Investment Model Variables, and Sexual Minority Stressors," *Partner Abuse* 2 (2011): 318.

109   **insecurely attached:** Dutton and Winstead, "Predicting Unwanted Pursuit," 576–81.

110   **The level of hurt, anger, frustration, resentment, loneliness, and jealousy all contribute to the likelihood of pursuit:** Ibid., 581, and Derlega et al, 318.

110   **A recent major personal loss:** In a telephone interview on February 14, 2014, forensic psychologist J. Reid Meloy said, "If you trace back in time what's happened to individuals who become very obsessed or have pursued someone to the point of stalking, you'll see a significant loss in their life in the weeks and months before the behavior began. You see a disrupted attachment, and the stalking becomes a way to defend against those feelings." His published research shows that 38 percent of female stalkers had suffered at least one major personal loss, usually a relationship, in the year prior to the stalking. Seventeen percent reported multiple losses, such as a relationship, finances, child custody, and a home. J. Reid Meloy and Cynthia Boyd, "Female Stalkers and Their Victims," *Journal of the American Academy of Psychiatry and the Law* 31 (2003): 216.

110   **unwanted pursuit is more likely to happen:** Research on same-sex unwanted pursuit shows that in addition to attachment style and level of investment in a relationship, "group-specific stressors (i.e., lifetime experiences with prejudice and discrimination among sexual minority individuals) uniquely predict unwanted pursuit behaviors." See Derlega et al, "Unwanted Pursuit in Same-Sex Relationships," 318. These findings are consistent with the "social ecology of marriage" theory, which holds that it is important to consider "macrosocietal forces and the ecological niche within which couples live" to fully understand how marriages work. See Ted L. Huston,

"The Social Ecology of Marriage and Other Intimate Unions," *Journal of Marriage and the Family* 62 (2000): 320.

110   **or grieving over the death of a loved one:** Fisher et al, "Reward, Addiction, and Emotion Regulation Systems Associated With Rejection in Love," 57.

111   **be overly tied up in having a man:** See Robin W. Simon and Anne E. Barrett, "Nonmarital Romantic Relationships and Mental Health in Early Adulthood: Does the Association Differ for Women and Men?" *Journal of Health and Social Behavior* 51 (2010): 178.

111   **it is a leading factor in suicide:** "Suicide Causes," Suicide.org, http://www.suicide.org/suicide-causes.html.

111   **heightens the risk of illness or death:** See Pekka Martikainen and Tapani Valkonen, "Mortality After the Death of a Spouse: Rates and Causes of Death in a Large Finnish Cohort," *American Journal of Public Health* 86 (1996): 1,087–93, http://www.ncbi.nlm.nih.gov/pmc/articles/PMC1380614/.

111   **the protest response is linked to our survival instincts:** Lewis et al, *A General Theory of Love*, 77–80.

117   **the brain's network for rage:** Helen Fisher writes that "love and hate are intricately linked in the human brain. The primary circuits for hate/rage run through regions of the amygdala downward to the hypothalamus and on to centers in the periaqueductal gray, a region in the midbrain. Several other brain areas are also involved in rage, including the insula, a part of the cortex that collects data from the internal body and the senses. But here's the key: the basic brain network for rage is closely connected to centers in the prefrontal cortex that process reward assessment and reward expectation. And when people and other animals begin to realize that an expected reward is in jeopardy, even unattainable, these centers in the prefrontal cortex signal the amygdala and trigger rage." Helen Fisher, *Why We Love: The Nature and Chemistry of Romantic Love* (New York: Henry Holt, 2004), 164.

5: Falling from the Stars

120   **More than half of the women in my online survey:** In response to the question "In your experience of unrequited love, what descrip-

tions best fit your reaction?," 55.72 percent of respondents checked "I felt like I was losing my mind"; 41.33 percent checked "I acted in ways I regret." The online survey was launched on May 1, 2010. Results were retrieved on March 19, 2014, at which point the survey had 261 complete responses. See http://www.lisaaphillips.com/survey/index.php?sid=24932&lang=en.

121 **(Shipman and Oefelein are now married . . .):** http://www.adventurewrite.com/about.html.

123 **"let-down period after the tremendous high of flying in space":** Andrea Lucia, "Letters Paint a Different Picture of Nowak," http://abclocal.go.com/ktrk/story?section=news/local&id=7118214.

123 **She was one of the rare ones who made it:** Except where otherwise noted, my account of Lisa Nowak comes from two sources: S. C. Gwynne, "Lust in Space," *Texas Monthly*, May 2007, 126–219; and Dianne Fanning, *Out There: The In-Depth Story of the Astronaut Love Triangle Case That Shocked America* (New York: St. Martin's Press, 2007).

124 **flooded with feeling:** Cupach and Spitzberg, *The Dark Side of Relationship Pursuit*, 105.

124 **lost her grip on reality:** Brizendine's quote is from C. W. Nevius, "When Love Goes Wrong—a Bizarre Mission," *The San Francisco Chronicle*, February 7, 2007, A1. Nowak ended up with a plea bargain that sentenced her to two days of time served and a year's probation. Her lawyer had planned to use an insanity defense in court on the basis of a psychiatrist's assessment that diagnosed bipolar disorder, obsessive compulsive disorder, Asperger's syndrome, and insomnia. Paul Siegel, an assistant professor of psychology at Purchase College, told *The Atlantic* that Nowak showed elements of antisocial personality disorder, which entails "disturbed patterns of thinking, feeling and behaving that come to the surface especially in relationships." People with this disorder often behave normally in everyday life but can be triggered by jealousy or other factors that reveal an instability underneath. See Ford Vox, "Lisa Nowak: Space Oddity," *Thealtantic.com*, February 17, 2011, http://www.theatlantic.com/national/archive/2011/02/lisa-nowak-space-oddity/71383/.

125 **triggering the urge to retaliate:** Forensic psychologist J. Reid Meloy said it was significant that Nowak was not pursuing the person

she was obsessed with. "If you can shift your fury toward a third object, you can preserve the fantasy toward the object you're pursuing. It's called triangulation. If you can blame a third party, you can still fantasize the other person loves you and wants to be with you. You can retain that special belief. You can believe the third party is interfering with that relationship." Telephone interview with Meloy, 2014.

127   **the redirection of feelings from a prior relationship:** Leonard H. Kapelovitz called transference "the inappropriate repetition in the present of a relationship that was important in a person's childhood." See Leonard H. Kapelovitz, *To Love and to Work: A Demonstration and Discussion of Psychotherapy* (Lanham, MD: Jason Aronson, 1977), 66. Transference was described first by Freud as an important process in psychoanalysis. The patient would experience transference with the analyst, who in turn could help her understand her feelings. Freud wrote: "The patient sees in [the analyst] the return, the reincarnation, of some important figure out of childhood or past, and consequently transfers on to him feelings and reactions which undoubtedly applied to this prototype." See Sigmund Freud, *An Outline of Psychoanalysis* (London: Hogarth Press, 1938), 125–26.

127   **lack of empathy for others:** "Narcissistic Personality Disorder Symptoms," http://psychcentral.com/disorders/narcissistic-personality-disorder-symptoms/.

131   **with the book open to the passage detailing his death:** Daniel Goleman, "Pattern of Death: Copycat Suicides Among Youth," *The New York Times*, March 18, 1987, http://www.nytimes.com/1987/03/18/nyregion/pattern-of-death-copycat-suicides-among-youths.html.

132   **losing him was portrayed as a reason to end her life:** Barbara T. Gates, "Suicidal Women: Fact or Fiction?" in *Victorian Suicide: Mad Crimes and Sad Histories, a Victorian Web Book*, http://www.victorianweb.org/books/suicide/07.html. "The Suicide" is published in *Forget Me Not: A Christmas and New Year's Present*, edited by Frederic Shoberl (London: R. Ackermann, 1827), 204–06.

132   **quoting a Bible passage from Corinthians:** 1 Corinthians 5:9–13: "But now I am writing to you not to associate with anyone who bears the name of brother if he is guilty of sexual immorality or greed, or is an idolater, reviler, drunkard, or swindler—not even to eat with such a one."

134   **loss of love is a common factor:** Suicide.org, a nonprofit suicide pre-
       vention organization, lists "the breakup of a relationship" as a cause of
       depression and states that "untreated depression is the number one
       cause for suicide." See Keven Caruso, "Suicide Causes," http://www
       .suicide.org/suicide-causes.html. A small study of suicide notes in
       India shows that a "disturbed love affair" was cited as a cause in 25
       percent of the forty suicide notes analyzed. Manjeet S. Bhatia, Satish
       Verma, O. P. Murty, "Suicide Notes: Psychological and Clinical Profile,"
       International Journal of Psychiatry in Medicine (2006): 36, 163–70.

135   **no single life event can be pinpointed as the only trigger for
       suicide:** Sonia Kutcher Chehil, *Suicide Risk Management: A Manual
       for Mental Health Professionals*, 2nd ed. (Hoboken, NJ: Wiley), 7.

139   **the other reads it as a buildup to romance:** Baumeister and Wot-
       man, *Breaking Hearts*.

6: The Gender Pass

146   **women are three times more likely than men to have been
       stalked:** According to the NIPSV survey, 16.2 percent of women and
       5.2 percent of men in the United States have experienced stalking vic-
       timization at some point in their lifetime. An estimated 10.7 percent
       of women and 2.1 percent of men have been stalked by an intimate
       partner during their lifetime. Michele C. Black et al, *The National In-
       timate Partner and Sexual Violence Survey: 2010 Summary Report*,
       2011, 1-2.

146   **believe that they or someone in their life would be harmed or
       killed as a result:** Ibid., 2.

146   **the gender disparity markedly diminishes:** "Research identify-
       ing men as the primary, and potentially more dangerous, perpetra-
       tors of stalking has not been without its exceptions. As noted above,
       gender differences fade in college sample studies of unwanted pur-
       suit behavior. In fact, in two studies with U.S. college students it
       was suggested that female perpetrators of unwanted pursuit engage
       in more mild aggressive stalking behaviors than men. . . . Another
       study . . . also found women engaged in more moderate levels of
       stalking behavior than men, and no gender differences were found

for severe stalking behavior." Amy E. Lyndon et al, "An Introduction
to Issues of Gender in Stalking Research," *Sex Roles* 66 (2012): 304.

146 **other forms of relationship violence and abuse:** Though crime
statistics show that women are usually the victims of relationship
aggression and men the perpetrators, community samples indicate
that women perpetrate a significant number of both "low-risk" and
more serious acts of violence against male partners. As with stalking,
the gender disparity fades significantly. See John Archer, "Sex Differences in Physically Aggressive Acts Between Heterosexual Partners: A Meta-analystic Review," *Aggression and Violent Behavior* 7
(2002), 339.

147 **compared to about a quarter of men:** Stacey L. Williams and
Irene Hanson Frieze's courtship behavior study at the University of
Pittsburgh showed that rival percentages of men and women used
surveillance behaviors (96 percent of men and 99 percent of women)
and mild aggression (27 percent of men and 22 percent of women)
during courtship. Mild aggression included trying to scare the person,
making threats, verbal abuse, and physical harm (both "slight" and
"more than slight"). After breakups, women were about as likely as
men to use intimidation (26 percent of men and 25 percent of women)
and somewhat more likely to use mild aggression (23 percent of men
versus 32 percent of women). See Williams and Frieze, "Courtship
Behaviors," 248–57. Leila Dutton's 2006 research on post-breakup
pursuit showed that female pursuers were more likely to monitor their
targets and more likely to physically hurt them. See Dutton, "Predicting Unwanted Pursuit," 575.

147 **the rate of women who stole or damaged property was twice
the rate of men:** In an analysis of three large studies of college
students and unwanted relationship pursuit tactics, 12 percent of
women reported they stole or damaged possessions compared to 6
percent of men. Eleven percent of women reporting doing physical harm, compared to 4 percent of men. Brian H. Spitzberg and
William R. Cupach, "What Mad Pursuit? Obsessive Relational Instruction and Stalking Related Phenomena," *Aggressive and Violent
Behavior* 8 (2003), 355.

147   **Female pursuers were just as likely as male pursuers to resort to severe violence, such as kicking and choking:** An Australian study published in *Sex Roles* in 2012 found that 28.8 percent of women who used repeated unwanted pursuit behaviors resorted to moderate violence such as slapping and grabbing, a rate approximately double that of male stalkers (15.5 percent). There was no significant gender difference in the rates of severe violence such as choking and kicking (16.9 percent of the males and 19.4 percent of the females). See Thompson, "Are Female Stalkers More Violent Than Male Stalkers?" 357. Even when stricter legal definitions of stalking are used, rates of violence among female stalkers have been comparable to that among males, and there is no evidence that the violence is any less serious or harmful when it's committed by female stalkers. See Meloy and Boyd, "Female Stalkers and Their Victims," 217.

147   **a sociocultural attitude that is more disapproving of male violence against women than female violence against men:** The study presented various scenarios to male and female relationship pursuers and found that they were more likely to see female violence against men as justified under certain circumstances than male violence against women. See Thompson, "Are Female Stalkers More Violent Than Male Stalkers?," 357–60.

152   **suffer from anxiety and shifts in their attitudes and personality:** Wigman, "Male Victims of Former-Intimate Stalking: A Selected Review," *International Journal of Men's Health* 8 (2009): 111–13.

152   **yet may be considered laughable when the roles are reversed:** Jennifer Langhinrichsen-Rohling, "Gender and Stalking: Current Intersections and Future Directions," *Sex Roles* 66 (2012): 421.

154   **"they should be ready to have a sexual experience with any woman, at any time":** Ibid., 421.

154   **female stalkers are not seen as being as much cause for concern as male stalkers:** Wigman, "Male Victims of Former Intimate Stalking," 109–10.

154   **rejecting a woman's love is, in the pagan world, a "sin against nature":** James Lasdun, *Give Me Everything You Have: On Being Stalked* (New York: Farrar, Straus and Giroux, 2013), 213.

156   **"accidentally (and dangerously) lead on a paranoid fantasist":**
        John Colapinto, "What Has He Done? On James Lasdun's Memoir,"
        Page-Turner blog, April 11, 2013, http://www.newyorker.com/online/
        blogs/books/2013/04/what-has-he-done-on-james-lasduns-memoir.html.

156   **"like Humbert Humbert, more complicit than innocent":** Jessica
        Freeman-Slade, "Like a Woman Scorned: On James Lasdun's Give
        Me Everything You Have," http://www.themillions.com/2013/03/like-
        a-woman-scorned-on-james-lasduns-give-me-everything-you-have
        .html.

156   **"while she remains alone, her novel unpublished, clearly
        very ill":** Nick Richardson, "Internet-Enabled," *London Review of
        Books*, April 25, 2013, http://www.lrb.co.uk/v35/n08/nick-richardson/
        internet-enabled.

156   **approaching his story with "an almost total lack of self-irony":**
        Jenny Turner, "Give Me Everything You Have: On Being Stalked—
        review," *The Guardian*, February 7, 2013, http://www.theguardian
        .com/books/2013/feb/07/give-me-everything-you-have-review.

159   **because society doesn't take female-on-male stalking seriously:**
        Langhinrichsen-Rohling, "Gender and Stalking," 422.

159   **more than 81 percent of the orders issued for male victims are
        violated, along with about 69 percent of the orders issued for
        female victims:** Christopher T. Benitez, M.D., Dale E. McNiel, Ph.D,
        and Renée L. Binder, M.D., "Do Protection Orders Protect?," *Journal
        of the American Academy of Psychiatric Law* 38 (2010): 376–85.

7: Crush

164   **"Part of Your World" is what's called the "I wish" song:** "Prom-
        ised Land," *This American Life*, originally aired on February 20, 2004,
        http://www.thisamericanlife.org/radio-archives/episode/259/transcript.

164   **marriageable young men and women might jostle against each
        other and meet:** See Julie C. Bowker, Sarah V. Spencer, Katelyn K.
        Thomas, and Elizabeth A. Gyoerkoe, "Having and Being an Other-
        Sex Crush During Early Adolescence," *Journal of Experimental Child
        Psychology* 111 (2012): 629.

166 **the distance he has said he wants:** Katie D. Anderson, "Teen Texting: The Ruin of Romance," *Huffington Post*, October 13, 2013, http://www.huffingtonpost.com/katie-d-anderson.

167 **would move on from these "homosexual attachments" as they grew older:** E. B. Hurlock and E. R. Klein, "Adolescent 'Crushes,'" *Child Development* 5 (1934): 63–80.

167 **Nearly every girl has had at least one crush by the age of fourteen:** Ninety-four percent of girls between twelve and fourteen report having had at least one crush. Kimberly D. Hearn, Ph.D.; Lucia F. O'Sullivan, Ph.D.; and Cheryl D. Dudley, M.A., "Assessing Reliability of Early Adolescent Girls' Reports of Romantic and Sexual Behavior," *Archives of Sexual Behavior* 32 (2003): 513–21.

167 **far more likely to have a crush than a relationship:** Fifty-six percent of middle-schoolers from four schools in suburban Buffalo had crushes, while 40 percent had an opposite-sex friend and 15 percent of students were in a relationship. Julie C. Bowker et al, "Having and Being an Other-Sex Crush During Early Adolescence," 363.

168 **the crush may transition into a mutual relationship:** Rivka Tuval-Mashiach, Sophie Walsh, Shirley Harel, and Shmuel Shulman, "Romantic Fantasies, Cross-Gender Friendships, and Romantic Experiences in Adolescence," *Journal of Adolescent Research* 23 (2008): 481–82.

168 **are linked with lower grades and standardized test scores:** Peggy C. Giordano, Wendy D. Manning, Monica A. Longmore, "Adolescent Romantic Relationships: An Emerging Portrait of Their Nature and Developmental Significance," *Romance and Sex in Adolescence and Emerging Adulthood*, ed. Ann C. Crouter and Alan Booth (Mahwah, NJ: Lawrence Erlbaum Associates, 2005): 140–41.

168 **much less likely than their peers to graduate from high school and enroll in college:** Serious daters go on dates at least once a week and/or have had sex. "Serious daters were much less likely to graduate from high school and enroll in college than were non-daters and moderate daters. While non-daters and moderate daters graduated from high school by the age of 20 at fairly high rates (85

and 86 percent respectively), only 73 percent of serious daters graduated from high school. . . . Similarly, only 59 percent of serious
daters had enrolled in college by the last wave of survey data collection, compared to 71 percent of moderate daters and 66 percent of
non-daters." Chung Pham et al, "Evaluating Impacts of Early Adolescent Romance in High School on Academic Outcomes," *Journal
of Applied Economics and Business Research* 3 (2013): 18.

168   **the greater the probability they will suffer from depression:**
Kara Joyner and J. Richard Udry, "You Don't Bring Me Anything but
Down: Adolescent Romance and Depression," *Journal of Health and
Social Behavior* 41 (2000): 369–91.

169   **dating relationships are their single greatest source of stress:**
Wendy D. Manning, Peggy C. Giordano, and Monica A. Longmore,
"Adolescent Dating Relationships: Implications for Understanding
Adult Intimate Unions," in *A Multidisciplinary Inquiry into Change
and Variation in Intimate Unions*, ed. L. Casper and S. Bianchi,
2008.

176–77 **in a 1992 essay on Beatlemania:** Barbara Ehrenreich, Elizabeth
Hess, and Gloria Jacobs, "Beatlemania: A Sexually Defiant Consumer
Subculture?" in *The Subculture Reader*, ed. Ken Gelder and Sarah
Thornton (London and New York: Routledge, 1997), 527.

177   **which might later be used to humiliate her:** Elizabeth Perle,
"THIS Is Why You Should F°°°ing Love Teenage Girls," *Huffington
Post*, October 24, 2013, http://www.huffingtonpost.com/2013/10/24/
why-i-fing-love-teenage-girls_n_4156383.html.

177   **there's no significant obligation or responsibility:** See Donald
Horton and R. Richard Wohl, "Mass Communication and Para-Social
Interaction: Observations on Intimacy at a Distance," *Psychiatry* 19
(1956): 215–29.

177–78 **"if you love me / then I'll never play Halo again":** Mike Lombardo, "Hey Molly," http://www.youtube.com/watch?v=ENZdTTXrdQ8.

178   **apology about his abusive relationship with an admirer:** Gavia
Baker-Whitelaw, "The Tom Milsom Abuse Scandal and YouTube's
Troubling Cult of Worship," *The Daily Dot*, March 14, 2014, http://
www.dailydot.com/fandom/tom-milsom-underage-sex-scandal/.

178   **manipulating underage girls into sending him sexually explicit photos and videos:** "YouTube 'Star,' 25, Jailed for Exchanging Explicit Images with Underage Female Fans," *Daily Mail*, March 1, 2014, http://www.dailymail.co.uk/news/article-2570619/New-York-musician-YouTube-star-25-imprisoned-five-years-exchanging-explicit-images-underage-female-fans.html.

179   **a push back against the manufactured conventions of teen sexuality:** Rachel Monroe, "The Killer Crush: The Horror of Teen Girls, From Columbiners to Beliebers," *The Awl*, October 5, 2012, http://www.theawl.com/2012/10/the-killer-crush-from-columbiners-to-beliebers.

181   **The movie wasn't distributed far beyond the film-festival circuit:** *Dear Lemon Lima* opened at one theater in Los Angeles. Yoonessi said she canceled a scheduled screening in Brooklyn because it was at a movie theater with a bar, where children were not allowed, and she considered the movie a "family film." The film was available for a while on Netflix and, at this writing, is available on Hulu. The film has had some international distribution. Telephone interview with Suzi Yoonessi on December 14, 2013.

183   *Legally Blonde,* **itself a fable about turning romantic rejection into empowerment:** Elle, the girlie and seemingly frivolous main character, is dumped by her boyfriend, who is about to start at Harvard Law School. She gains admission to the program in the hope of winning him back. She loses interest in the boyfriend and becomes a brilliant law student.

8: Primal Teacher

185   **some kind of transcendent "union of the soul" relationship:** Clare R. Goldfarb, "Female Friendship: An Alternative to Marriage and the Family in Henry James's Fiction?" *Colby Quarterly* 26 (1990), http://digitalcommons.colby.edu/cgi/viewcontent.cgi?article=2804&context=cq.

188   **"changed my life for the better":** In response to the multiple-choice question "How did your most significant experience of unrequited

love affect your life?," 32.10 percent of the women who filled out my online survey responded, "It changed my life for the better." Forty percent responded, "It changed my life for the worse," and 14 percent responded, "It did not really change my life." See http://www .lisaaphillips.com/survey/index.php?sid=24932&lang=en.

188 **"the lover is forced to notice what is missing":** Jacqueline Wright, "Bittersweet Eros," Jung Society of Atlanta newsletter, Fall 2004, http://www.jungatlanta.com/articles/fall04-bittersweet-eros .pdf.

189 **yearning, longing, or regret for "that which is elsewhere":** Page du Bois, *Sappho Is Burning* (Chicago: University of Chicago Press, 1997), 29.

189 **"I am and dead—or almost / I seem to me":** Anne Carson, *Eros the Bittersweet* (Princeton, NJ: Princeton University Press, 1986), 13.

189 **and enjoy being inspired:** Aron et al, "Motivations for Unreciprocated Love," 787.

190 **should last only as long as the feeling of love:** Wollstonecraft and Imlay came together, agreeing on theories about "the importance of freedom and immorality of maintaining a tie once feeling had ceased to sanction it." Claire Tomalin, *The Life and Death of Mary Wollstonecraft* (New York: Signet Classic, 1974), 179.

191 **she wrote from Paris in 1795:** Janet Todd, ed., *A Wollstonecraft Anthology* (Bloomington: Indiana University Press, 1977), 242.

192 **followed by reassurances that she was overcoming the pain:** After spotting a wild pansy called Heart's Ease on the shores of Sweden, she wrote, "a cruel remembrance suffused my eyes, but it passed away like an April shower." Ibid., 147.

192 **discredit Wollstonecraft's feminism (as some modern critics have done):** See Susan Eilenberg, "Forget That I Exist," *London Review of Books*, November 20, 2000, http://www.lrb.co.uk/v22/n23/ susan-eilenberg/forget-that-i-exist.

192 **the "creature of feeling and imagination":** Todd, ed., *A Wollstonecraft Anthology*, 185.

192 **"keep me no longer in suspense!—Let me see you once more!":** Ibid., 253.

193   **"We reason deeply, when we forcibly feel":** Ibid., 168.

193   **that might have silenced her forever:** My description of Wollstone-craft's relationship with Imlay and its impact on her work is based on Claire Tomalin's *The Life and Death of Mary Wollstonecraft* (1974) and Janet Todd's *A Wollstonecraft Anthology*. Additional resources include Christina Nehring's account of Wollstonecraft's life in *A Vindication of Love*, 176–92.

193   **the passionate expressiveness that would distinguish *Jane Eyre* and *Villette*:** Lucasta Miller, *The Brontë Myth* (New York: Knopf, 2001), 124.

193   **a book that stunned its original audience with its emotional frankness:** Ibid., 14–16.

194   **A nine-year-old girl wonders why, if the email author says he loves Calle, is he leaving her?:** Henry Samuel, "Conceptual Artist Dumped by Email Gets Revenge on Ex-love," *The Telegraph*, April 25, 2008, http://www.telegraph.co.uk/news/1903952/Conceptual-artist-dumped-by-email-gets-revenge-on-ex-lover.html.

194   **sue her for invasion of privacy, then changed his mind:** Giovanni Intra, "a Fusion of Gossip and Theory," http://www.artnet.com/magazine_pre2000/index/intra/intra11-13-97.asp.

195   **portray the desire of two lovers to merge into one being:** Western tradition has from Plato's symposium the tale of the two missing halves reuniting. The Persian poet Rumi tells us that "lovers do not find each other; they are in each other." This concept can have a spiritual dimension, with devotional writings that are indistinguishable from love poetry, as in the lavishly sensual Song of Songs. It doesn't matter, Zeki argues, whether we can say for sure whether the Song of Songs is about desire for God or for another human. What matters is that the brain concept of ideal love is so lofty that it counts for both divine and profane love. Zeki, *Splendors and Miseries of the Brain*, location 2762.

195   **reinforcing the concept of union in love:** Ibid., location 2349-2393.

197   **Her sister-in-law, Susan Gilbert?:** Steven Cramer, "Emily Dickinson, 'I cannot live with You,'" *The Atlantic*, April 14, 1999, http://www.theatlantic.com/past/docs/unbound/poetry/soundings/dickinson.htm.

197   **"If I am constantly working, my relationships fail":** Mark Jefferies, "The Real Adele," *The Mirror*, February 15, 2012, http://www

.mirror.co.uk/3am/celebrity-news/the-real-adele-grammy-sensation-talks-685087, and James Montgomery, "Adele Says *21* Has People Thinking 'I'm Sort of a Manic-Depressive,'" *MTV News*, February 18, 2011, http://www.mtv.com/news/articles/1658345/adele-21.jhtml.

198   **thought to be related to emotion and reward in decision-making:** Zeki, *Splendors and Miseries of the Brain*, location 1085.

198   **found near the center of the brain:** T. Ishizu and Semir Zeki, "Toward a Brain-Based Theory of Beauty," PLoS ONE 6 (2011), http://www.plosone.org/article/info%3Adoi%2F10.1371%2Fjournal.pone.0021852.

198   **primal, dopamine-fueled rush of desire:** Brain scan studies of love-struck men and women, conducted by Lucy Brown, Helen Fisher, and colleagues, showed activity (increased blood flow, as detected on an fMRI scan) in the Ventral Tegmental Area, as discussed in chapter three, and the Caudate Nucleus. "Ventral Tegmental Area and Caudate Nucleus," Brain Maps LLC, accessed July 7, 2014, http://theanatomyoflove.com/the-results/the-brains-reward-system/ventral-tegmental-area/.

198   **outsider identity, which rejection reinforces, nurtures their ability to innovate:** Art Markman, "Ulterior Motives," *Psychology Today*, August 16, 2013, http://www.psychologytoday.com/blog/ulterior-motives/201308/does-rejection-make-you-creative.

199   **"which gave me the joys which Love withheld":** Isadora Duncan, *My Life* (New York: Horace Liveright, 1928), ebook at http://www.gutenberg.ca/ebooks/duncani-mylife/duncani-mylife-00-h-dir/duncani-mylife-00-h.html.

203   **protagonists driven by unrequited love to suicide, insanity, or depression:** Joke Hermes, "Sexuality in Lesbian Romance Fiction," *Feminist Review* 42 (1992): 49–66.

9: Letting Go

209   **called what I went through *starvation*:** "Limerence for a particular LO does cease under one of the following conditions: *consummation*—in which the bliss of reciprocation is gradually either blended

into a lasting love or replaced by less positive feelings; *starvation*—in which even limerent sensitivity to signs of hope is useless against the onslaught of evidence that LO does not return the limerence; *transformation*—in which limerence is transferred to a new LO." Tennov, *Love and Limerence*, 255.

210   **a number of therapeutic approaches rooted in cognitive behavioral therapy:** See Frank Tallis, "Crazy for You," *The Psychologist* 18, February 2005, 74.

211   **After the treatment, glucose metabolism in that area decreased, along with the symptoms:** See Jeffrey M. Schwartz, "First Steps Toward a Theory of Mental Force: PET Imaging of Systematic Cerebral Changes After Psychological Treatment of Obsessive-Compulsive Disorder" in *Towards a Science of Consciousness III: The Third Tucson Discussions and Debates*, ed. Stuart R. Hameroff, Alfred W. Kaszniak, and David J. Chalmers (Cambridge, MA: Massachusetts Institute of Technology, 1999): 111–21. The book Schwartz wrote with Rebecca Gladding, *You Are Not Your Brain: The 4-Step Solution for Changing Bad Habits, Ending Unhealthy Thinking, and Taking Control of Your Life* (New York: Penguin, 2011), details for a popular audience his program for coping with "deceptive brain messages," which he defines as "any *false or inaccurate* thought or any *unhelpful or distracting* impulse, urge, or desire that takes you away from your true goals and intentions in life (i.e., your true self)."

215   **"All that was once so beautiful is dead":** Conrad Aiken, "Discordants," *Turns and Moves and Other Tales in Verse* (New York: Houghton Mifflin, 1916), 24.

218   **nearly half of all convicted stalkers overall reoffend:** The study describes the application of a six-month treatment program to a sample of twenty-nine individuals, fourteen of whom completed treatment. Treated offenders were significantly less likely to reoffend with another stalking offense (zero of fourteen) compared to treatment dropouts (26.7 percent) or to published recidivism data (47 percent). Barry Rosenfeld, Michele Galietta, Andre Ivanoff et al, "Dialectical Behavior Therapy for the Treatment of Stalking Offenders," *International Journal of Forensic Mental Health* 6 (2007): 95.

222 **the same pharmacological treatments for addiction might apply to people suffering from the loss of love:** Caroline M. Hostetler and Andrey E. Ryabinin, "Love and Addiction: The Devil Is in the Differences: A Commentary on 'The Behavioral, Anatomical and Pharmacological Parallels Between Social Attachment, Love and Addiction,'" *Psychopharmacology* 224 (2012): 27–29.

224 **The caring presence of other people:** Geoff MacDonald and Mark R. Leary, "Why Does Social Exclusion Hurt? The Relationship Between Social and Physical Pain," *Psychological Bulletin* 131 (2005): 207.

Selected Bibliography

Ackerman, Diane. *A Natural History of Love.* New York: Random House, 1994.

Adams, Jeffrey M., and Warren H. Jones, eds. *Handbook of Interpersonal Commitment and Relationship Stability.* New York: Kluwer Academic/Plenum Publishers, 1999.

Alighieri, Dante. *La Vita Nuova.* Translated by Barbara Reynolds. New York: Penguin Books, 2004.

Argov, Sherry. *Why Men Love Bitches: From Doormat to Dreamgirl.* Avon, MA: Adams Media, 2000.

Aron, Arthur, Elaine N. Aron, and Joselyn Allen. "Motivations for Unreciprocated Love." *Personality and Social Psychology Bulletin* 24 (1998): 787–96.

Baily, Beth L. *From Front Porch to Back Seat: Courtship in Twentieth-Century America.* Baltimore: Johns Hopkins University Press, 1988.

Baumeister, Roy F., and John Tierney. *Willpower: Rediscovering the Greatest Human Strength.* New York: Penguin Books, 2011.

Baumeister, Roy F., and Sara R. Wotman. *Breaking Hearts: The Two Sides of Unrequited Love.* New York: Guilford Press, 1992.

Behrendt, Greg, and Liz Tuccillo. *He's Just Not That Into You: The No-Excuses Guide to Understanding Guys.* New York: Simon & Schuster, 2004.

Bergner, Daniel. *What Do Women Want?: Adventures in the Science of Female Desire.* New York: Ecco Press, 2013.

Black, M. C., et al. *The National Intimate Partner and Sexual Violence Survey: 2010 Summary Report.* Atlanta, GA: National Center for Injury Prevention and Control, Centers for Disease Control and Prevention, http://www.cdc.gov/ViolencePrevention/pdf/NISVS_Report2010-a.pdf.

Bloch, R. Howard. *Medieval Misogyny and the Invention of Western Romantic Love*. Chicago: University of Chicago Press, 1992.

Bolt, Rodney. *The Impossible Life of Mary Benson: The Extraordinary Story of a Victorian Wife*. New York: Atlantic Books, 2012.

Bowen, Elizabeth. *The Death of the Heart*. New York: Alfred A. Knopf, 1938.

Brontë, Emily. *Wuthering Heights*. Edited by William M. Sale. New York: W. W. Norton, 1972, 1963.

Brontë, Charlotte. *Villette*. New York: Everyman's Library, 1992.

———. *The Professor*. New York: Penguin Books, 1989.

Buss, David M. *The Dangerous Passion: Why Jealousy Is as Necessary as Love and Sex*. New York: Free Press, 2000.

Carcopino, Jérôme. *Daily Life in Ancient Rome: The People and the City at the Height of the Empire*, 2nd ed. New Haven: Yale University Press, 2003.

Carson, Anne. *Eros the Bittersweet*. Princeton, NJ: Princeton University Press, 1986.

Cervantes, Miguel de. *Don Quixote*. Translated by Edith Grossman. New York: HarperCollins, 2005.

Cheever, Susan. *Desire: Where Sex Meets Addiction*. New York: Simon & Schuster, 2008.

Crouter, Ann C., and Alan Booth, eds. *Romance and Sex in Adolescence and Emerging Adulthood*. Mahwah, NJ: Lawrence Erlbaum Associates, 2005.

Cupach, William R., and Brian H. Spitzberg. *The Dark Side of Relationship Pursuit*. Mahwah, NJ: Lawrence Erlbaum Associates, 2004.

Dow, Leslie Smith. *Adèle Hugo: La Misérable*. Fredericton, NB: Goose Lane Editions, 1993.

Dowling, Colette. *The Cinderella Complex: Women's Hidden Fear of Independence*. New York: Summit Books, 1981.

Faludi, Susan. *Backlash*. New York: Crown, 1991.

Fanning, Dianne. *Out There: The In-Depth Story of the Astronaut Love Triangle Case That Shocked America*. New York: St. Martin's Press, 2007.

Felson, Richard B. *Violence and Gender Reexamined*. Washington, D.C.: American Psychological Association, 2002.

Ferrand, Jacques. *A Treatise on Lovesickness*. Translated and edited by Donald A. Beecher and Massimo Ciavolella. Syracuse, NY: Syracuse University Press, 1990.

Fielding, William J. *Strange Customs of Courtship and Marriage*. New York: New Home Library, 1942.

Findling, Rhonda. *Don't Call That Man!: A Survival Guide to Letting Go*. New York: Hyperion, 1999.

———. *Don't Text That Man!: A Guide to Self-Protective Dating in the Age of Technology*. New York: New York City Girl Publishing, 2012.

Fisher, Helen. *Why We Love: The Nature and Chemistry of Romantic Love*. New York: Henry Holt, 2004.

Forward, Susan, and Craig Buck. *Obsessive Love: When It Hurts Too Much to Let Go*. New York: Bantam, 1991.

Frieze, Irene Hanson, ed. *Sex Roles: A Journal of Research* 66, no. 5–6 (2012).

Galen. *On Prognosis*. Translated by Vivian Nutton. Berlin: Akademie-Verlag, 1979. http://cmg.bbaw.de/epubl/online/cmg_05_08_01.html.

Gaylin, Willard, and Ethel Person, eds. *Passionate Attachments: Thinking About Love*. New York: Free Press, 1988.

Geher, Glenn, and Scott Barry Kaufman. *Mating Intelligence Unleashed: The Role of the Mind in Sex, Dating, and Love*. New York: Oxford University Press, 2013.

Goethe, Johann Wolfgang von. *The Sorrows of Young Werther*. Translated by Burton Pike. New York: Random House, 2004.

Harevon, Gail. *The Confessions of Noa Weber*. Brooklyn, NY: Melville House Publishing, 2009.

Hatem, M. Abdel-Kader. *Life in Ancient Egypt*. Los Angeles: Gateway Publishers, 1976.

Hendrick, Susan S., and Clyde Hendrick. *Romantic Love*. Newbury Park, CA: Sage Publications, 1992.

Highsmith, Patricia. *The Price of Salt*. New York: W. W. Norton, 1984.

Jacquart, Danielle, and Claude Thomasset. *Sexuality and Medicine in the Middle Ages*. Translated by Matthew Adamson. Princeton, NJ: Princeton University Press, 1988.

Jankowiak, William, ed. *Romantic Passion: A Universal Experience?* New York: Columbia University Press, 1995.

Josephson, Matthew. *Stendhal or The Pursuit of Happiness*. New York: Doubleday & Company, 1946.

Jung, Emma. *Animus and Anima*. Woodstock, CT: Spring Publications, 1957.

Kapelovitz, Leonard H. *To Love and to Work: A Demonstration and Discussion of Psychotherapy*. Lanham, MD: Jason Aronson, 1977.

Kipnis, Laura. *Against Love: A Polemic*. New York: Pantheon, 2003.

Kraus, Chris. *I Love Dick*. Los Angeles: Semiotext(e), 2006.

Kundera, Milan. *Slowness*. Translated by Linda Asher. New York: HarperCollins, 1996.

Lasdun, James. *Give Me Everything You Have: On Being Stalked*. New York: Farrar, Straus and Giroux, 2013.

Lewis, Thomas, Fari Amini, and Richard Lannon. *A General Theory of Love*. New York: Random House, 2000.

Lystra, Karen. *Searching the Heart: Women, Men, and Romantic Love in Nineteenth-Century America*. New York: Oxford University Press, 1989.

McMillan, Tracy. *Why You're Not Married . . . Yet: The Straight Talk You Need to Get the Relationship You Deserve*. Ballantine Books, 2013.

Meloy, J. Reid, ed. *The Psychology of Stalking: Clinical and Forensic Perspectives*. San Diego: Academic Press, 1998.

Messud, Claire. *The Woman Upstairs*. New York: Alfred A. Knopf, 2013.

Miller, Lucasta. *The Brontë Myth*. New York: Alfred A. Knopf, 2001.

Munck, Victor C., ed. *Romantic Love and Sexual Behavior: Perspectives from the Social Sciences*. Westport, CT: Praeger, 1998.

Neely, Carol Thomas. *Distracted Subjects: Madness and Gender in Shakespeare and Early Modern Culture*. Cornell University Press, 2004.

Nehring, Christina. *A Vindication of Love: Reclaiming Romance for the Twenty-first Century*. New York: Harper, 2009.

O'Shea, Samara. *Loves Me . . . Not: How to Survive (and Thrive!) in the Face of Unrequited Love*. New York: February Books, 2014.

Robb, Graham. *Victor Hugo*. New York: W. W. Norton, 1997.

Schwartz, Barry. *The Paradox of Choice: Why More Is Less*. New York: Ecco Press, 2003.

Schwartz, Jeffrey M., and Rebecca Gladding. *You Are Not Your Brain: The 4-Step Solution for Changing Bad Habits, Ending Unhealthy Thinking, and Taking Control of Your Life*. New York: Penguin, 2011.

Sittenfeld, Curtis. *Prep*. New York: Random House, 2005.

Staël, Germaine de. *Delphine*. Translated by Avriel H. Goldberger. Rockford, IL: Northern Illinois University Press, 1995.

Summerscale, Kate. *Mrs. Robinson's Disgrace: The Private Diary of a Victorian Lady*. New York: Bloomsbury, 2012.

Stendhal. *On Love*. Translated by Philip Sidney Woolf and Cecil N. Sidney Woolf. Mount Vernon, NY: Peter Pauper Press (1916).

———. *The Life of Henry Brulard*. Translated by Catherine Alison Phillips. New York: Alfred A. Knopf, 1939.

Sternberg, Robert A., and Michael L. Barnes, eds. *The Psychology of Love*. New Haven, CT: Yale University Press, 1988.

Tallis, Frank. *Love Sick: Love as a Mental Illness*. New York: Thunder's Mouth Press, 2004.

Tennov, Dorothy. *Love and Limerence: The Experience of Being in Love*. Lanham, MD: Scarborough House, 1999.

Tomalin, Claire. *The Life and Death of Mary Wollstonecraft*. New York: Signet Classic, 1974.

Todd, Janet, ed. *A Wollstonecraft Anthology*. Bloomington, IN: Indiana University Press, 1977.

Tuchman, Barbara W. *A Distant Mirror: The Calamitous 14th Century*. New York: Random House, 1987.

Waldman, Adelle. *The Love Affairs of Nathaniel P*. New York: Henry Holt, 2013.

Wack, Mary Frances. *Lovesickness in the Middle Ages: The Viaticum and Its Commentaries*. Philadelphia: University of Pennsylvania Press, 1990.

Weber, Jill P. *Having Sex, Wanting Intimacy: Why Women Settle for One-Sided Relationships*. Lanham, MD: Rowman & Littlefield, 2013.

Wharton, Edith. *The House of Mirth*. New York: Charles Scribner's Sons, 1976.

———. *The Age of Innocence*. New York: Charles Scribner's Sons, 1968.

Whitehead, Barbara. *Why There Are No Good Men Left: The Romantic Plight of the New Single Woman*. New York: Broadway Books, 2003.

Williams, Tennessee. *A Streetcar Named Desire: A Play in Three Acts*. Sewanee, TN: University of the South, 1981.

Zeki, Semir. *Splendors and Miseries of the Brain: Love, Creativity, and the Quest for Human Happiness*. West Sussex, UK: John Wiley & Sons, 2009.

Index

About the Author

LISA A. PHILLIPS, a journalism professor at the State University of New York at New Paltz, has published articles and essays in the *New York Times*, the *Boston Globe*, Psychologytoday.com, and other publications. A former award-winning radio reporter, she has worked at public radio stations across the country and contributed stories to NPR and Marketplace. She is also the author of *Public Radio: Behind the Voices*. Phillips lives in Woodstock, New York, with her husband and their daughter.

Lisaaphillips.com
Twitter.com/lisaamyphillips